INDIANA UNIVERSITY

SCHOOL OF MEDICINE
Department of Family Medicine

*This book is given to you
compliments of the
Department of Family Medicine
and the Franciscan St Francis
Health Family Medicine Residency*

Franciscan ST. FRANCIS HEALTH
FAMILY MEDICINE RESIDENCY PROGRAM

Family Practice Stories

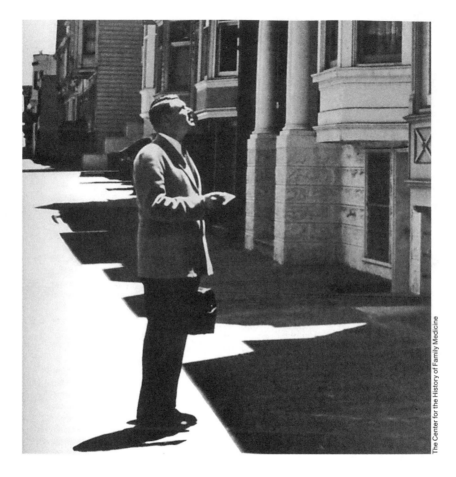

The Center for the History of Family Medicine

This book was supported by

The Max Feldman, M.D. Memorial Fund, Indiana Academy of Family Physicians Foundation

Family Practice Stories Book Fund, Indiana Academy of Family Physicians Foundation

Family Medicine Philanthropic Consortium, American Academy of Family Physicians Foundation

The Center for the History of Family Medicine, American Academy of Family Physicians Foundation

Family Practice Stories

Memories, Reflections, and Stories of Hoosier Family Doctors of the Mid-Twentieth Century

WRITTEN AND EDITED BY

Richard D. Feldman, MD

Indiana Historical Society Press | 2013

© 2013 Indiana Historical Society Press

This book is a publication of the
Indiana Historical Society Press
Eugene and Marilyn Glick Indiana History Center
450 West Ohio Street
Indianapolis, Indiana 45202-3269 USA
www.indianahistory.org
Telephone orders 1-800-447-1830
Fax orders 1-317-234-0562
Online orders @ http://shop.indianahistory.org

Chapter 2 is excerpted from *Doc: Memories from a Life in Public Service* by Otis R. Bowen with William Du Bois Jr. (Bloomington: Indiana University Press, 2000) and is used with permission.

The paper in this publication meets the minimum requirements of American National Standard for Information Sciences—Permanence of Paper for Printed Library Materials, ANSI Z39. 48–1984

Feldman, Richard D.
Family practice stories : memories, reflections, and stories of Hoosier family doctors of the mid-twentieth century / written and edited by Richard D. Feldman, MD.
    pages cm
Includes index.
ISBN 978-0-87195-314-8 (cloth : alk. paper)
1. Physicians (General practice)—Indiana—Anecdotes. 2. Physicians—Indiana—Biography. 3. Medicine, Rural—Indiana—Anecdotes. 4. Indiana—Biography. I. Title.
R153.F45 2013
610.92—dc23
                    2013008545

To the memory of my father, Max Feldman, MD, and the family doctors of that "Greatest Generation," the physicians who created the modern specialty of family medicine.

Contents

Foreword

Soothing Medicine

Georgia Perry

There were times during the two years I worked on this project when I needed a doctor. Not a doctor of today, one who could diagnose a sore throat, an allergy, or infection, but a doctor of yesterday. One who would sit with me and just let me know that things were going to be okay. Who knew the value in that kind of care? Thanks to the Indiana Academy of Family Physicians and to this project, I've had the good fortune of meeting about a dozen such doctors.

The day I got the first phone call about working as an interviewer and contributing writer on this project, I was a couple months out of college. I lived in Bloomington, Indiana, for what would be one last summer before moving on to Chicago and eventually Portland, Oregon. When I got the call, I was walking with my friends back from the limestone quarries, where we spent the day sunbathing and jumping off forty-foot cliffs into clean green water. I was wearing a red swimming suit and brown Chuck Taylor sneakers. The sun was setting golden brown as we walked along a dusty dirt road back to the parking lot of a big church where we'd left my car. I was twenty-two years old. Plans were forming to go out for ten-cent buffalo wings at Mother Bears'

Pizza when we got back to town. My phone rang.

I spoke to Paul Arnold, a local writer I knew who was involved with the Academy's project for a short time. He thought I would be a good fit. I listened to him on the phone from across the church's parking lot while my friends tried to talk a cop out of issuing us a trespassing ticket. This was where my college days and my new, adult life intersected— here in the fading sunlight of this parking lot. I had a job, it seemed.

Paul gave me the Academy's phone number and suggested I call Doctor Richard Feldman, who was spearheading the project. I borrowed a pen from the cop to scrawl the number down on my hand. I still don't remember if we got a ticket that day.

The majority of the doctors I interviewed for this project invited me into their homes and spoke with me in person. I would wake in the morning and set off on adventures all over the state: two, three hours away sometimes. Nervous about traffic and getting lost in winding subdivision neighborhoods, I usually arrived in the doctors' towns about a half hour early. I remember these preinterview half hours fondly as they were spent perusing the aisles of quaint local groceries and soaking up the small-town life, foreign to me in my Indianapolis upbringing. In Delphi I bought a baby food-sized can of Vienna sausages, in Tell City a packet of homemade walnut fudge. In New Albany I stopped at the local drugstore for a soda and with ballpoint pen on the ladies' bathroom wall drew a heart and wrote the name of the boy I still loved, who was from there and who had recently left me.

Later, during the interviews, the doctors would tell me about how they'd lived in the same towns for decades and got recognized, thanked, and asked questions everywhere they went. They often heard, "Do you remember me? You delivered me!," and would have to explain that the person speaking to them looked a little different than the day they were born. I always asked the doctors if they ever got tired of that sort of thing. None of them did.

After the interviews I would leave town and notice that everything looked different. The roads transformed into the dirt roads the doctors spoke of that led them to their patients' homes in the country. The sidewalks became the paths they took to get to little offices in the center of town, then walked back on to have dinner with their families, before returning for evening office hours.

The doctors I spoke to are men and women who spent forty plus years working six days a week, taking midnight phone calls to make house calls in the backcountry of Indiana, sometimes given no more directions than, "Our house is the one that looks like a cereal box." They didn't have heaters in their cars, so they brought house cats along with them to keep their laps warm on those middle-of-the-night drives. They volunteered hour after hour as team physicians for local high school sports teams, taking no payment besides season tickets to root on the local boys and girls. The majority are still involved in a volunteer capacity at clinics across the state, and a few still maintain their practices. A doctor in Princeton looked me square in the eye over a bowl of chili at his favorite diner and told me he fully intends to keep working until he drops dead in his office, just like his uncle did.

When I started this project, I came from a world of studio apartments and overdue electric bills. While working on this project, a collection agency hunted me down for the $54 I owed to the Monroe County Public Library for a delinquent paperback. I am not even listed in the 2010 census because I lived in so many different apartments that year. Graduating in the middle of an economic recession sent me into a spiral of panic. I developed breathing difficulties and lay awake most nights past the witching hour. What on earth was I doing, I wondered, pursuing a career as a writer?

Hearing the doctors' stories soothed me more than any medication that could have been prescribed. From them, I learned what it meant to commit to a purpose worth caring about. I learned about patience, and I learned about accepting mistakes and learning from them. Many doctors spoke stoically about patients they could not help or lives they regretfully could not save early on in their careers—patients they would have been able to save later, with the technology and experience they gained over the years. They were sad for losses but resigned to be forgiving of themselves looking at the big picture. They spoke about the importance of listening to others, of placing a hand on a patient, and listening to a heartbeat. They told me stories of life and death, and of the simple things that make it all worthwhile.

After all their decades—combined, centuries—of listening to patients, now it is the doctors' turn to share. I hope you will read this collection and enjoy it. I hope when you cannot sleep at night or you're scared or confused or lonely, you can pick it up and find comfort in its pages. I hear that the golden age of medicine is gone, replaced with insurance forms, expensive machines, and stricter and stricter office hours. But the golden age of medicine does not have to exist exclusively in the realm of practicing physicians. I hope this collection inspires you, like it has inspired me, to listen patiently, forgive ourselves, and never underestimate the healing power of listening to someone's heart.

Preface

Family Practice Stories is an initiative of the Indiana Academy of Family Physicians and the Indiana Academy of Family Physicians Foundation. The idea for the book was not mine, but percolated up through the organization beginning around 2001. The early project involved a very small group led by one of my former academic colleagues, Judith Monroe, MD, who at the time was the program director of the Saint Vincent Family Medicine Residency Program in Indianapolis. The group collected a few stories (that unfortunately could not be located and are not included in this book) to test the feasibility of the endeavor. Other pressing obligations, however, took them away from this work. I was then only peripherally involved with the project, but I felt strongly that capturing and preserving stories from elder family physicians was too important an endeavor to let languish. So in 2004 I felt compelled to see it through to completion; with Monroe's blessing, I became the new captain of the project.

The book is almost entirely an oral history. I knew that collecting the stories would be time and labor intensive, and that it would require a collaboration of a group of individuals assisting me by traveling around Indiana to collect the transcripts of the forty-eight elder Hoosier family doctors who agreed to be interviewed. I gathered a little team that included a resident physician in my residency program at Franciscan Saint Francis Health in Indianapolis, an Indianapolis journalist, and several journalism students at Indiana University. Finally, I enlisted a few individuals to write specific essays for Part One of the book. It was tedious work and at times I felt discouraged. Could we actually get all these doctors interviewed? Would the stories be interesting, charming, and alluring enough to become a book worthy of publishing? Would it appeal to the general public as well as the medical community?

The history, values, and traditions of family medicine date back more than 150 years in America, but the modern specialty of family medicine was fashioned by the emulation of the philosophical underpinnings of the general practitioners of the mid-twentieth century. They are truly the specialty's elder statesmen. It is my belief that this book will, indeed, not only resonate professionally with family doctors and other physicians, but also with all individuals who affectionately remember the family doctor who cared for them as a child or sometime during their lives.

The family doctors contained in this work were all Hoosiers; however, they are representative of all family physicians of that era wherever they may have lived. They could have practiced in New York or Nebraska, California or Arkansas, or any other state. Their stories are the same; there is a commonality to the values they reveal.

Writing and editing this book has been a journey. My only regret is that this project did not occur a decade earlier because there are so many notable family physicians that were already gone by the time the interviews for the book were initiated.

I am proud of my involvement in this project because this book accomplishes our goal of preserving the golden age of family medicine, not so much through a rote written history, but through storytelling. Some stories are humorous, some are serious, some are touching, and some are sad. But every story is important because by reading these stories we can come to know the essence of that era in medicine. There are lessons to be learned. And besides, everyone loves a good story.

Richard Feldman, MD
July 2013

Acknowledgments

This book was collaboration. The author wishes to acknowledge Judith Monroe, MD, who promoted the original concept for this book and to express his gratitude to the following individuals who provided their assistance in its development. Contributing authors Georgia Perry; Andrew Campbell, MD, and Gus Pearcy, for their important contributions and for conducting many of the physician interviews; contributing authors Jeff De Wester, MD, Deborah Allen, MD, and Nick Hrisomalos, MD, for their valuable involvement; Ashley Lichtenbarger, S. Ryan Brown, and Paul and Carol Arnold, who conducted several additional physician interviews; my wife Becky Feldman for her detailed review of my manuscript; Indiana Academy of Family Physicians staff members Deeda Ferree and Missy Lewis, who provided their gracious assistance in many aspects of this endeavor; Dawn O'Neil and Elizabeth Hudson for their assistance in creation of the biographical sketches; Jenny Kirby, who transcribed many of the interviews; Amy Bova for her assistance in creating the final submission copy to the Indiana Historical Society Press; and Clarence Clarkson, MD, Edwin Stumpf, MD, Robert Kopecky, MD, and Wayne Hardin, MD, for their participation. Also to Indiana University Press for granting permission to reprint portions of *Doc: Memories from a Life in Public Service*. Thanks also to Ray E. Boomhower and Kathy Breen, editors with the Indiana Historical Society Press, and Amberly Howe and David Turk from the IHS's Preservation Imaging Department for scanning the photographs used in the book.

Editor's Note

Whenever possible, the original interview transcripts were used for the stories that follow with some narrative comments from the author. Because of differing characteristics of some individual transcripts and interview situations, and because some interviews were with relatives of deceased physicians, differing styles of composition were utilized to best create the story.

The transcripts were edited only to add clarity and conciseness and to improve the flow and readability of the story. In a few instances, minor changes were made to disguise the identity of a patient.

The terms "general practice," "family practice," and "family medicine" were considered interchangeable depending on the era and context in which the term was used.

Introduction

Richard D. Feldman, MD

"Our family doctor is retiring the first of November. What a surprise. One never thinks about his doctor leaving, always taking it for granted that he will be there. And he was, whenever we needed him—in the middle of the night or during his working hours. He always took the time to listen and advise.

"From measles to mumps, sprained knees to broken bones, heart attacks to surgery, he was ever present, reassuring and helpful. We never worried. . . . Some would say it was his job, his profession, his duty to be there. We look at it differently. We weren't a dollar sign—we were people in need.

"He was and is a good family doctor. . . . we will miss you, sir."

This letter, which captures the essence of the traditional family doctor, was written to the editor of the *South Bend Tribune* in 1983. It's about my father, Max Feldman. A family doctor in South Bend, Indiana, for nearly forty years, he passed away in 2003 at the age of ninety-three. I believe he was exemplary of the traditional family doctor that these words capture so wonderfully; the physician who many have experienced in their lives and fondly regard. I am proud to be my

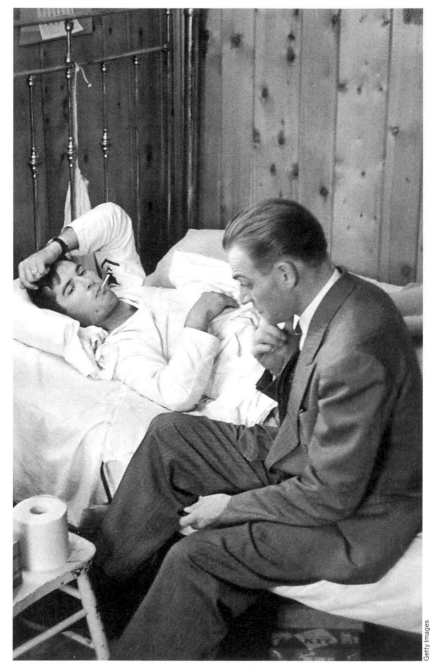

When family doctors made house calls, they never knew what they might find. It could be everything from routine ailments to heart attacks.

father's son, but he was not unique. He was only one example of so many fine family doctors of his time.

My father was a person of great character and determination. He was devoted to his family and to his profession, and he served as a primary role model in my life and in my career as a family physician. His life in many respects is not only the story of America but also the story of family medicine.

His family came to America through Ellis Island in 1920 seeking a new life free from poverty and anti-Semitism. As a child, his entire family lived in a fourth-floor, single-room tenement apartment on Delancy Street in Manhattan. He worked his way through school and did well. Dad was one of the most intelligent people I have ever known, but because of the quota system in those days that limited the number of Jewish students admitted to American medical schools, he was unable to attend medical school in the United States.

He returned to Europe to attend medical school at Konigsberg, Germany, and Basil, Switzerland. My father was a courageous individual who defied the Nazis in 1933 as a young medical student. He endured the Great Depression and was valiant as a medical officer at Pearl Harbor on that infamous day on December 7, 1941. Typical of that Greatest Generation, his character and values as a person and a doctor were shaped by such experiences. It was from this generation of family doctors, our founding fathers, from which the contemporary specialty of family medicine grew.

After graduating from medical school in 1937, my father completed two years of rotating internships in New York City hospitals. I remember dad telling me that during his first internship he lived at the hospital and made just fifteen dollars a month. After his training, as did most new physicians at that time, he went into the general practice of medicine. He called himself a general practitioner. In those days, it was not a demeaning term or a term that signified something less than what you were. My dad was kind, modest, and unassuming in nature. Possessing a wisdom that came with experience and understanding people, he was always pragmatic in his approach to situations and to life. He was known as one of the brightest and best family physicians in South Bend. He displayed an incredible fund of medical knowledge and always amazed me with his understanding of the physiologic basis of disease processes. He only consulted when he reached the limits of his abilities. He read his journals every night, he saw his patients in the office and in their homes, and he took care of them in nursing homes and in the hospital, even some who were critically ill. He delivered babies, set many of his patients' fractures, and performed tonsillectomies.

Today, the concepts and core values of the discipline of family medicine are incorporated into standardized formal residency training and board certification. But no family medicine residency programs existed in those earlier days. The principles of comprehensive and continuous personalized patient care came to him and other general practitioners of his generation by experience and sensitivity to the needs of their patients. They knew their patients well and were committed to their communities. Especially in small towns, they were among the most respected individuals and were considered as trusted friends by their patients. These physicians were humbled and honored to be invited into the lives of their patients. They seemed to intuitively understand, as William Osler once said, "It is more important to know the patient than to know what disease the patient has."

The formal specialty of family medicine was created from these best traditions and attributes of general practice. But as well-known family physician and educator, Nick Zervanos, MD, once recounted, it was created out of necessity. The over specialization of medicine in postwar America reached a point that threatened the very survival of the general practitioner. It was at a time when medical knowledge, research, and technology were exponentially expanding, stimulating the development of medical specialties. The GI Bill helped pay for medical school and up to four years of residency training, so the number of specialty residencies grew swiftly and the ranks of specialists swelled (there were no general practice residencies).

Graduating medical students flocked to the specialties that offered greater prestige, larger incomes, and, with the explosion of medical

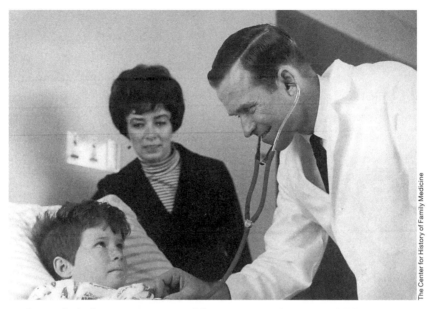

A pleasing bedside manner was one of the prerequisites for a successful family doctor.

knowledge, the security of mastering only a limited area or organ system. Many believed general practice was simply on its way out. General practitioners returned from the war finding it difficult to obtain hospital and surgical privileges in the new age of specialized medicine. Although held in esteem by their patients, general practice physicians, especially in metropolitan areas, felt disrespected by the larger medical community. The family doctor was fading away.

In reaction to these threats, generalists rallied in support of their profession. The American Academy of General Practice was founded in 1947 for the purpose of garnering political voice, protecting hospital privileges, preserving the practice of general medicine and encouraging new physicians to enter the field, promoting continuing medical education and research, and maintaining high standards of medical practice for its members. General practice continued to struggle, but the new organization was successful in enhancing the public's recognition of the general practitioner's role in medicine.

Yet, the lack of family physicians extended to every segment of our nation. The loss of the trusted adviser and compassionate counselor who cared for every problem for everyone in the family from birth to death was lamented by the American people. The time-honored general practitioner, who took the opportunity to talk and develop ongoing relationships with his patients, advocated for them, and coordinated their health care, was still highly desired.

Society was changing. Health insurance was made more available to American workers, but there was increased concern for the availability of medical services for the poor and elderly. The vision was for a health-care system based on all patients having a medical home with a personal physician. It was evident to government, academic and organized medicine, health-related foundations and associations, the press, and the public that something had to be done to satisfy this societal need; thus, the new specialty of family medicine was born.

The creation of the American Board of Family Practice in 1969 established family practice as the twentieth medical specialty and reversed the trend away from primary care by bolstering the stature of the family physician within American medicine. The first three-year residency training programs in family practice were established that year. The American Academy of General Practice was renamed the American Academy of Family Physicians in 1971. Today, patient visits to family doctors account for the largest proportion of doctors' office visits.

Family physicians do not have a monopoly on what's good in the medical profession. Family physicians are not better than other doctors, but they are different. They continue to be the heart and soul of medicine. More than any other specialty, family doctors humanize the health-care experience. Focusing their attention on the person, not just the disease, they are driven by the need to make people whole and develop relationships over generations with the patients and families under their care. Ask any family doctor what makes his or her profession rewarding and fulfilling and that's what they will tell you. That's what family physicians do. I present the family doctor as an idyllic figure in American culture, but I believe it is real and can be validated by anyone who has had a long-term, comforting, and reassuring relationship with their family doctor.

A few years ago the discipline of family practice underwent an organized, in-depth self-evaluation called the Future of Family Medicine Project. The initiative's goal was to identify its core attributes and develop a strategy to transform and renew the specialty to meet the needs and expectations of the contemporary American public. Even the name of the specialty was changed from "family practice" to "family medicine." The final report from the project concluded that family practice must reformulate itself and reconstruct its place in medicine to assure future public confidence. But the core values of family medicine remained unchanged. It's not surprising, because they define our very identity and our uniqueness. It is simply who we are.

The medical world has changed radically in the last twenty-five years, and the family physician has not been immune to these developments. Medicine is again overspecializing, fueled by corporate interests and a market-driven health-care system. It is a paradigm that promotes the expansion of procedural medicine and specialty practices squeezing the last and most profitable dollars from the health-care system. Primary care physicians are increasingly employed by health-care corporations that judge and pay them mainly on the basis of productivity. Our reimbursement system is not designed to reward spending time with patients to counsel and educate, or to promote health and prevent disease, or to develop the necessary therapeutic relationship by knowing the patient as a person. Medicine is becoming increasingly depersonalized as a system largely dominated by a business ethic. Patients can easily become widgets.

I was recently reminded of the thought that we see the future by standing on the shoulders of the past. No matter how medicine changes, the future will belong to those physicians who deliver caring, humanistic, and compassionate care. That's what family doctors do. And that's why family medicine will hold a central role in the inevitable transformation of the American health-care system in the new millennium.

Family Practice Stories is a collection of tales told by, and about, Hoosier family doctors practicing in the middle of the last century. It celebrates that time in America considered by many to be the golden age of generalism in medicine. It is a book about a time gone by—a time when professionalism, the art of medicine, and the art of healing were at their zenith. It was a simpler paternalistic time in medicine that conjures up Norman Rockwell's familiar archetypal images of the country family doctor. Writing this book was an important endeavor to accomplish, for it captures these stories before they are lost forever.

The book is divided into two sections. The first is a collection of reflective essays on various subjects. Some reflections are written by individuals who participated in interviewing these older doctors, some are written by invited essayists, and others are the perspectives of the doctors themselves concerning medicine and their careers. The second section is the heart of the book that contains a large collection of stories told by, and about, Hoosier family physicians that practiced during this era. The stories are specific episodes in their careers. Each story stands by itself as a single chapter taken from the original transcripts of the interviews.

May this book be a source of pride for family physicians and portray to the public who we are, what we do, what we believe in, and the proud traditions from which we come. May it serve as a remembrance of the lives of these family doctors, their style of medicine, and how they touched their patients and communities.

We're family physicians. We are different. We have a story to tell.

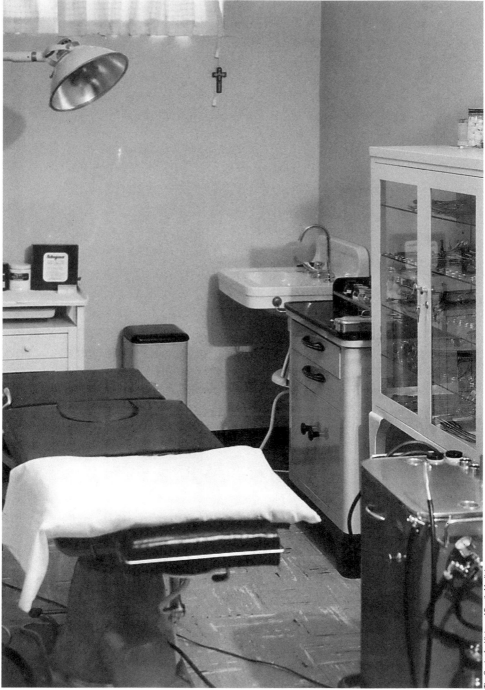

Part 1
Reflections

1

A Tribute to the Family Doctor

Gus Pearcy

"Shot?!" The four-year-old boy's ears and eyebrows perked as if they were on rockets. Shots were the absolute worst thing in the world; much worse than the throbbing earache that prompted the call to the doctor in the first place.

It was the mid-1960s and Frank Beardsley, MD, was making a standard house call to the home of my grandparents, Crawford and Bernadine Barker, in Frankfort, Indiana. Doctor Beardsley had delivered me a few years earlier and now was appearing as the mean ol' doc who wanted to stick a poor waif with a syringe. It was not a role he enjoyed.

I apparently thought the only chance I had was to run. So I did—all over a two-story home that was decorated for the Christmas holiday. I was caught on the stairway attempting to hurdle the banister. I cried. Doctor Beardsley aimed the needle at my buttocks and jabbed but could barely look because of the fear and pain he knew he was causing. It was necessary to be "cruel to be kind." It was actually a prerequisite of medicine over the centuries.

I lived and felt fine just in time for a fabulous Christmas. Doctor

Beardsley went on to deliver several more babies and shots of penicillin while medicine continued to evolve into the complicated science it is today. But the art remains as constant as the caduceus.

The metamorphosis of medicine in the last century is truly remarkable. From the advent of life-giving antibiotics to the immunization against scourges such as polio and the eradication of smallpox, medicine continues to discover more ways to make life worth living. Increasing numbers of medical professionals are specializing in one area of the body or one discipline of care, perhaps at the cost of the human side of medicine. Science is an uncaring beast consuming massive meals of factoids to spit out concrete conclusions. The casualty is a caring bedside manner valiantly kept alive by the family physician. The evolution of medicine has been good for the body, but the family doctor was always good for peace of mind. Eventually, science will be able to quantify what members of the Indiana Academy of Family Physicians have ascribed to for more than fifty years already: Good care begins with a caring attitude.

This book celebrates the last century of comprehensive medical care from the family doctor's perspective. It is a testament to house calls, baby deliveries, miracles, and the dedication that many of us have felt from our family physicians. It also serves as a reminder that while advances in medicine are saving thousands of lives every day, health care is still dependent upon the "care" to make it work.

Conducting some of the interviews for this book, I have talked to family physicians who were crowned with the ability to ease worried minds and foster goodwill in thousands upon thousands of patients. Their stories will help restore faith in the art of "bedside" manner. Technology has overcome many of the impediments to a full and productive life, but caring always will be a vital component to a patient's well-being.

Success magazine founder Orison Swett Marden wrote, "There is no medicine like hope, no incentive so great, and no tonic so powerful as expectation of something better tomorrow." These are what the steady hand, the confident smile, and the knowledgeable nod of the family physician bring to the patient and the patient's loved ones.

Our tribute to the work of the family physician is a debt of gratitude to the art of medicine.

2

A Country Doc

Otis R. Bowen, MD

The late Otis R. Bowen, MD, was undoubtedly the most esteemed family physician in Indiana. He is remembered not only as a Hoosier country doctor but also for his distinguished political career.

Bowen was born near Rochester, Indiana, in 1918. He attended Indiana University receiving an AB in 1939 and a MD in 1942. He served an internship in 1942 at Memorial Hospital in South Bend, Indiana. From 1943 to 1946, he served in the Medical Corps of the U.S. Army in the Pacific theater, reaching the rank of captain. He was with the first wave of allied troops going ashore in the invasion of Okinawa in 1945. Upon his return from World War II, he practiced in his hometown of Bremen, Indiana, until 1972. During this time, he began his political career as the elected coroner of Marshall County, Indiana.

Bowen, a Republican, served in the Indiana House of Representatives from 1956 to 1958 and again from 1960 to 1972. He was Speaker of the House from 1967 to 1972. He was elected to two terms as governor of Indiana from 1972 to 1980.

After completing his second term as governor, Bowen accepted a clinical professorship in the Department of Family Medicine at the IU School of

Medicine, where he taught until he was appointed by President Ronald Reagan in 1985 as Secretary of Health and Human Services. Following his term, Bowen retired from medicine and public life in 1989.

During his tenure as governor, Bowen worked on Indiana's landmark malpractice reform act that he signed into law in 1975. Indiana's law was the first in the nation and has served as a national model over the years.

With a family to feed, I needed to begin a practice. Beth and I looked for a place where I could be a country doctor and still be reasonably close to good hospitals and consultative services. We also wanted a good place to settle down and rear a family.

We visited many areas. We chose Bremen because of its proximity to South Bend's Memorial and Saint Joseph hospitals and Mishawaka's Saint Joseph Hospital, and because I knew the specialists in South Bend. Beth and I also liked Bremen's attractive homes, well-maintained businesses, excellent schools and parks, and many churches.

Bremen's only doctor, Homer Burke, was returning to the medical mission field. (Doctor Earl Cripe, also back from the service, started practice in Bremen the same day I did.) I bought the old house that Doctor Burke had used as his office, purchased the equipment, furniture, and medical supplies, and bought medical instruments from a Bourbon physician's widow. The office had a large waiting room, two examining rooms, a medicine room, and a restroom on the main floor and a delivery room upstairs. I hired an office nurse, Bernice Crittenden, a secretary-receptionist, Lydia Heuberger, and an on-call OB nurse.

I also bought a small home, earlier the office of Doctor Wallace Buchanan, who did not return to Bremen after the war. Once remodeled, it became our first home. As I began practice, my goal was to be the most caring family physician possible. If I was available and conscientious and didn't gouge patients, I assumed that I would be as busy as could be.

I saw my first patient, Fred Lehman, in the evening on Memorial Day, 1946. His was an easy poison ivy case. My $1.50 charge for the office call included a bottle of calamine lotion. I kept fees at $1.50 for a few months then slowly increased them until office visits were $5 and house calls were $7 by 1972. My initial fee for prenatal care, including the mother's six week postdelivery checkup, her baby's first month checkup, their night in the office's upstairs delivery room, and a nurse's services, was $35. By 1972 it reached $75. One reason I could keep fees so low was that malpractice insurance was only $15 a year. However, that cost soon zoomed rapidly upward.

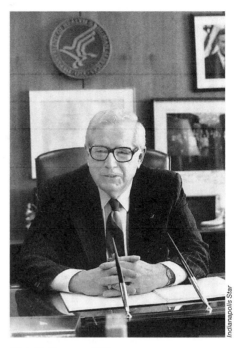

Otis R. Bowen, MD

I was busier than I'd ever imagined. My practice covered a twenty-five to thirty-mile radius from Bremen north to Lakeville, Mishawaka, and South Bend, east to Nappanee, west to Tyner, Walkerton, Koontz Lake, and LaPaz, and south to Bourbon, Argos, and Plymouth.

Medical school gave me book knowledge and theory. The internship helped me apply that knowledge. In my first months of practice, I became my own teacher. The practice of medicine jibed with my medical school teachings, but we had not been taught how to run an office, schedule appointments, do consultations, write job descriptions, hire personnel, handle payroll, deal with tax issues, and handle "hurt feelings and little jealousies" among office personnel. We also got little advice in school on how to integrate ourselves into our communities or keep up with new medical techniques and medicines.

My practice dealt mostly with upper respiratory and gastrointestinal illnesses, earaches, sore throats, arthritis, and common communicable diseases—"three-day" and "old fashioned" measles, mumps, and chickenpox. In medical school, internship, and the military, I seldom saw such illnesses. I removed skin tumors, did "T&A's" (tonsil and adenoid surgeries) and "D&C's" (dilation and curettage surgeries), delivered babies, and did episiotomies in the delivery room. I assisted with surgeries on patients I referred to surgeons. I repaired lacerations of every kind and took care of simple fractures.

I handled 80 to 90 percent of all cases, referring the rest to specialists. I routinely made referrals on cases involving appendectomies, gall bladder removal, tumors other than skin tumors, complicated fractures, and medical or pediatric diagnostic problems. If I sensed that patients or relatives were overly anxious, or when patients did not respond to accepted treatment measures, I made referrals.

Referrals can be defensive. If patients sense that a physician is competent and caring, there are minimal legal dangers in practicing in a small town. In other settings, even with friendly patients and capable physicians, the dangers are greater. If a parent, spouse, or child is ill, it's a threat when the family member in charge says, "I don't care what it costs. Get my wife (or child or parent) well." Doctors then must do expensive tests that won't show anything but will prove that the physician did everything possible.

On average, I delivered about ten babies a month, or about 120 a year. Over twenty-five years in practice, I estimate that I delivered 3,000 babies. Long before it was common, I allowed husbands in the delivery room, warning them to sit or leave if they became lightheaded or dizzy. Few had to sit. Husbands and wives were thankful for this opportunity to share a special family moment, the birth of a child.

My office's upstairs delivery room had a labor bed, a delivery table, and supply cabinets. Unless patients wanted to go elsewhere, I delivered babies there, as Doctor Burke had, until Bremen Hospital became a reality. After staying overnight, my patients were carried down the narrow stairway on a stretcher by Johnny Siefer and Ernie Goss, employees of Huff Funeral Home, and taken by ambulance to the home of either Mrs. Jennie M. Bartels or Mrs. Francis A. Maurice. Those ladies cared for them until ten days were up. It was a far cry from today's immediate ambulation.

My typical day started at 6:30 a.m. with a quick breakfast at the town café (Beth was busy getting the kids off to school.) After hospital rounds and house calls, I started office calls at 9:00 a.m. An emergency room call, a delivery, or seriously ill walk-in patient could put us behind. If we ran late, our secretary called the next patient. Morning and afternoon times were left open for catch-up. Over the noon hour, I worked in a house call or two, had a quick lunch, and returned to the office to see patients with appointments until roughly 6:00 p.m. After one or two more house calls, I went home, ate, listened to the news, and went to bed. Often I had a night house call or two.

I categorized patients in four groups—those with appointments, work-ins, walk-ins, and sneak-ins. We tried to stay on schedule for those with appointments. Work-ins were told to come in but were promised no specified time. They usually had high temperatures or were otherwise acutely ill. We saw them between appointments or by scheduling them in open appointment times. Most walk-ins were quite sick, and we cared for them the best we could. A typical "sneak-in" was a mother with an appointment who brought three kids along and said, "While I'm here, would you look at them too?" If we had time, we did. If we didn't and they were not acutely ill, we suggested that they come back.

Patient loads depended upon the time of year. In a flu epidemic, if we had two or three imminent deliveries at the same time, if there was a major accident, if there was snow and ice on the ground, or if it was excessively hot or cold, we had more patients. My average daily patient load was about four patients on hospital rounds (not counting OB cases), four or five house calls, including those at night, and about twenty-five office patients.

I considered house calls an integral part of my practice. This was particularly true for Amish patients. Bringing a mother or two or three sick children to my office in a buggy was especially difficult for them. I could do a better job in my office, but an examination at home was better than none at all, and it was infinitely better than dragging a sick infant or an ill elderly patient out in bad or wintry weather.

For crippled or hypertensive older patients, I scheduled house calls—monthly, every other month, or every third month. Once these future house calls were noted in my appointment book, patients knew they could expect me at that time on that day. Serving twenty to thirty nursing home patients took half a day every month. Usually nursing home patients' greater susceptibility to illness added an emergency call or two a week.

I drove myself on most house and emergency calls. If I was extremely tired and admitted it after an urgent call in the middle of the night, Beth drove. Nora Sausman, who lived alone two blocks away, came on short notice to stay with our children. At times, house calls were difficult. On one to an Amish lady's home up a long, muddy lane, my car got stuck. My patient's husband quickly pulled me out—with a team of horses.

In northern Indiana, snowdrifts and blocked roads are common in winter. In my car's trunk, I carried boots, gloves, a heavy coat, salt, and a scoop shovel. In the worst part of winter, I had chains on my tires. One night I got stuck near Buford Rowe's home, three or four miles out in the country. He probably heard me revving the car's motor, because I had just started shoveling when he came with his tractor. Occasionally, perhaps trying to save a fee for an office call, people caught me at the post office or church or on the street and asked a medical question. If my patience was shorter than normal, my answer was: "Undress right now and I'll check you."

Elderly patients were my pets. It took longer to examine them and deal with their problems, but they appreciated the attention. Elderly persons who accepted aging as a time to expect slowing and aches and pains and not to expect miracles were my least difficult patients. Babies were no problem except for their over-anxious parents. Children from two to eight years of age were less apt to be cooperative.

I am a great fan of the Amish people, a group of honest, friendly, tidy, hardworking, generous, religious folks. They handle most things themselves. If a family member is ill and can't afford needed care, all chip in. When an Amish family's barn burns, they put up another one in days. In twenty-five years of practice, I had only one Amish patient on welfare, an elderly alcoholic man.

The Amish do not use electricity, but most have indoor plumbing. They do not own cars, but some hire a vehicle and driver for a vacation or visit. They have no telephones, but often use the closest neighbor's in an emergency.

My Amish patients were no different than other patients. When they called, however, I knew they were really sick, because their call meant that their home remedies had failed. Amish children were good patients—either well disciplined or very shy—and they never misbehaved in my office or their homes.

Before Bremen had a hospital providing obstetrical care, Amish women had babies at home. If an Amish man called or an Amish kid showed up at my home or office and said, "Come on out, Mom's sick," I knew I should take along my obstetric bag. After we got the hospital, the Amish were a bit reluctant to use it for deliveries. Once they started doing so, word quickly spread about how nice it was to have a baby there. Amish women still wanted to go home twenty-four to forty-eight hours after giving birth. At the time, I was reluctant to let that happen. In retrospect, they were ahead of the times.

The Amish became and remain ardent Bremen Community Hospital supporters. Each year, the hospital auxiliary stages a fund-raising barbecue. The Amish supply wonderful homemade pies, attend in significant numbers, wait tables, and help clean up.

Amish patients never paid me on the spot for a Sunday call, but they were always at the door the next morning to pay.

My patients included two more than a hundred years old. I did an appendectomy on a ninety-year-old lady. I cared for five generations in one family and delivered children to three generations of several families. I enjoyed taking care of ministers, some of whom came back for physicals after moving away, possibly because I never charged them.

I once delivered the seventeenth child for one family. They couldn't afford to pay, and I didn't ask for anything. Being good people and wanting to do something, they left a chicken in a gunnysack in our garage. Wouldn't you know it, I ran over the chicken.

When medical problems or minor surgery was involved, I sent

patients to Bremen Hospital. For major surgery, patients went to Saint Joseph Hospital in Mishawaka or Memorial Hospital in South Bend. I always asked patients and their families where they wanted to go. Most preferred our local hospital, where they were babied and where relatives could visit easily. Even after major surgeries at Mishawaka or South Bend, patients often transferred back to Bremen in two to three days. Before the local hospital opened, patients needing hospitalization went to South Bend, Mishawaka, or Plymouth. Keeping patients in Bremen saved time for patients, families, and doctors. There are hundreds of interesting anecdotes from my quarter-century in the practice of medicine, and a few memorable ones.

One patient, Delbert Snyder, broke his back and severed his spinal cord in a fall off a wagon. I cared for him as an intern at South Bend Memorial, and then cared for him for many more years after returning from the service.

I remember a family across the tracks that included about five children, the youngest a girl I had just delivered. Three or four days after she and her mother got home from the hospital, I was called to come see the baby. Her towheaded five-year-old brother met me at the door and said, "Come on in, Doc. My baby sister won't nurse and poops all the time." (I've substituted "nurse" and "poops" for his actual words.)

I once was called to the house of a young farmer, Richard Baker, whose illness had baffled physicians, including a South Bend specialist. When he was lying down, his blood pressure was okay. When he sat up, he fainted and his blood pressure dropped. He suffered dizziness. I had seen only one case as an intern, but Addison's disease came to my mind immediately. Tests showed that my hunch was correct. Cortisone treatments improved his condition dramatically. Since Addison's is a chronic disease, he had to stay on the medication. I felt proud that I made a rare diagnosis after others had failed.

I delivered a set of twins whose combined weight was fourteen pounds. Wondering if that was a record, I checked the State Board of Health. The twins' birth weight was the second heaviest in state history.

Occasionally, people conclude what they want. I carefully explained to the family of a farmer who had suffered a coronary occlusion, commonly called a heart attack, what had happened and what it meant. After I was through, a daughter said, "Well, thank God; I thought he'd had a heart attack." A delightful little old lady who hadn't seen a doctor much came to me. Her daughter had told her that she would have to undress for the examination. We gave her a hospital-type gown to wear. When I came into the exam room, I saw that she had put on her pajamas.

One of my Amish patients was an eight- or nine-year-old boy with the biggest adenoids and tonsils I've ever seen. When he took a breath, he literally snorted. I convinced his parents that he needed a T&A surgery. Two weeks later, my young patient came to my office for another reason. "Doc," he said, "I'm sure glad you took out my tonsils. Now when we play hide-and-seek, they can't find me."

The case of JoAnn Senff, born with a hole in the septum of her heart, was unique. She faced certain death without surgery. At age fourteen or fifteen, when she was close to that point, we contacted Doctor Harris B. (Harry) Shumacker Jr., a heart surgeon and the chair of the Department of Surgery at the IU School of Medicine. He said immediate surgery had to be done.

JoAnn had the rarest blood type—A negative. Before surgery, we needed thirteen pints of that type blood. I obtained an A-negative donor list from the Red Cross Blood Bank, called those on it, and asked them to help. Some lived as far as a hundred miles away from Indianapolis, but no one turned me down—an example of the abiding goodness of people.

The surgery was successful. JoAnn needed a pacemaker, but she married and had two children, who I helped deliver by Caesarean. She died at about age forty-five, before her children were grown, but had a longer, fuller life than otherwise would have been possible.

Within two years after coming to Bremen, my practice had grown so much that I was working eighty-hour weeks and had a house call or delivery most nights. I built a new office building in 1948, but it was obvious that what I needed most was help. Marshall E. Stine, a graduate of Washington Medical School in Missouri, joined my practice the next year. After Doctor Stine went into the service, Doctor Cecil R. Burket of nearby Wakarusa joined me in practice. As a South Bend Memorial intern, he relieved me a weekend or two a month and was familiar with my practice. He and his wife, Bernice ("Bunnie") Burket, a nurse, stayed at our home and used my office to see patients when he relieved me. On Doctor Burket's first day, I had a 104-degree temperature and tonsillitis, and he had to go it alone.

After Doctor Stine's return, we formed a three-man family practice group. Doctors Stine and Burket were very competent, compassionate physicians. The three of us were remarkably compatible. (Doctor Stine passed away on April 14, 1999, in Naples, Florida. For the hospital newsletter, I prepared a eulogy that said in part: "From close personal experience, I can say that Marshall was a master at his job. He had the old standing virtues. He was well informed, conscientious, gentle, and gracious. He was polite, attentive, and a good listener—qualities that made him a good counselor to his patients. He was organized, considerate, and reliable. He deserves to be called a true professional—one dedicated to his God, his family, his community, his friends, and his patients.")

As our practice evolved, I added another nurse, a business manager, and a person to transcribe information from a recording device into which we dictated each patient's complaints, what our exam showed, and what we prescribed. This helped us keep our records current. Our business manager, William Helmlinger, served all three physicians. When I later left the group, he continued with Doctors Burket and Stine until retirement.

The group practice gave each of us time off. I took Wednesday afternoons, Doctor Burket Thursdays, and Doctor Stine Fridays. Every third weekend I was on call. Every third weekend I worked until Saturday noon and was on second call—the back-up physician—for emergencies or major problems. Every third weekend I was off from Friday night to Monday morning. The doctor on full duty covered "walk-ins" at 11:00 a.m. Sundays. When they learned that a doctor was available then, a few patients who should have been to the office earlier or could have waited took advantage. Not many did, and the doctor on call could see all the patients needing treatment on a weekend in two hours.

When Doctor Jack Schreiner came to Bremen to practice solo, the community had five doctors and good medical coverage. All five were about the same age and retired about the same time. Several physicians saw that as an opportunity and the community now has seven fine doctors in their thirties and forties.

My legislative service later required me to spend large blocks of time away from Bremen. These absences were unfair to my colleagues. In 1964 I sold my office to Doctors Burket and Stine, put an office in the basement of my home at 304 North Center Street, and resumed solo practice. During legislative sessions, my former colleagues covered for me.

In solo practice, I made my own appointments and was able to keep on time. When patients called, I asked about their ailment. If they had a sore throat, I scheduled them for ten minutes. If the patient was a talkative older lady needing a physical and Pap test, I allowed an hour. Dressing and undressing—and talking—took a lot of extra time.

The 1965 Palm Sunday tornadoes, which took 139 lives in Indiana and caused massive property destruction, created medical problems that far exceeded any I had ever experienced except during the war. About 2,000 people were injured statewide.

Mrs. Calvin Grise of Wyatt was brought to our hospital on a door. A two-by-six-inch splintered board had sliced into her abdomen. Miraculously, it had not gone into the abdominal cavity, but had kind of split the skin over the abdomen. She also had a broken leg. It took us hours to get the wound cleaned and sutured and to set the fracture.

Bremen Community Hospital doctors and staff handled their share of tornado-related medical problems. Comparatively speaking, our hospital was busier than the larger South Bend hospitals, which saw about 100 patients. We saw about thirty.

Events had an unsettling quality at times. I've always found it difficult to accept the deaths of young people, particularly those in auto accidents. While coroner, I was called to the west edge of Bremen, where an accident had taken the lives of two boys. Both were about sixteen and barely able to drive. Just before the accident, they had tried to coax their good friend, our son Tim, into going with them. Tim knew he couldn't stay long after school without reporting home, so he didn't go. Beth and I were forever grateful that he didn't.

Dealing with a patient's death is difficult. I tried to be sympathetic and understanding and made it a point to explain to family members what had happened. I went to the funeral home to pay my respects and to create another opportunity for the family to talk with me about their loved one. It's a tightrope walk. Being too emotional reduces one's ability to think and act professionally. Being totally unsympathetic looks (and is) cold and hard-hearted. Later, after losing loved ones of my own at too early an age to cancer, I came to think that—despite my best efforts—I might not have shown enough warmth and empathy. There is no greater trauma than losing those who occupy special niches in our lives.

I practiced in Bremen from 1946 to 1971. Running for and serving as governor later kept me from practicing. I've never regretted the fact that I did not specialize or practice in an urban area. Being a small town family doctor involves a special, satisfying, and uplifting relationship. In Bremen, I was more than a physician. I was a friend, neighbor, fellow Kiwanian, band booster, and sports enthusiast like other townspeople. I no longer practice in Bremen, but I still enjoy a special relationship with its wonderful people.

Medicine has changed a great deal in the fifty-plus years since I started practice. I don't know when I realized that doctors must be both competent and compassionate. It's not enough to have competence without compassion, or vice versa. At some point, I also realized that some of the worst medical students were the best doctors because of the art of their practice, and some of the best medical students were poor doctors because patients saw their minimal charisma as cold and unfeeling.

Specialization and government intervention depersonalized medicine. Other factors, including shallow media coverage, make people expect the impossible—medical miracles on demand all the time. When things go wrong, people now sue, even if the doctor made an honest mistake or the problem was outside his control. Such developments negatively impact the practice of medicine.

The federal health care programs, Medicare and Medicaid, have been boons to patients and to some degree economic boons for doctors. However, the paperwork and occasionally goofy regulations associated with the two programs make doctors feel that someone is looking over their shoulder. This has altered the doctor-patient relationship and increased the cost of medicine.

Doctors had more charitable hearts when I practiced. Certainly, money counted, but not like it does now. At that time, doctors seemed more willing to donate time to free clinics for the poor.

Despite the negatives, we see new and different miracles on an almost daily basis. I personally know many compassionate doctors. Fifty-plus years after I first began practice in Bremen, I still believe that the practice of medicine is the noblest of all professions.

Antibiotics are the biggest change in medicine in my lifetime. Sulfanilamide was a miracle drug when I graduated from medical school. I first heard about penicillin when Winston Churchill became ill in Africa or the Mediterranean, was treated with penicillin, and made a miraculous recovery. Penicillin also gave the armed services a one-shot cure for gonorrhea. The tetracyclines followed. One after another, new antibiotics came along. Today's doctors have an array of infection-fighting drugs. There also are new medicines for hypertension, vaccines, and diagnostic tools like CAT scans and MRIs; advances in transplant surgery, renal dialysis, and laboratory procedures; new treatments for cancer, open heart surgery, birth control pills, and so on.

The first cases of AIDS undoubtedly developed in the sixties, but we did not know about them until later. We now seem to be at the start of the journey toward a cure.

In short, the changes we have seen in medicine in these last fifty years are a revolution, the end of which is not in sight.

Immense changes in medicine also have taken place in Bremen in my fifty-plus years there. A large crowd turned out when Bremen

Community Hospital celebrated its fiftieth anniversary on June 16, 1997. The open house came seventeen days after my nephrectomy—removal of a cancerous kidney. Though still a bit under the weather, I had to be present, because I was there at the beginning. Doctors Stine and Burket and I were the speakers.

In 1943, Mr. and Mrs. William Myers started a nursing and convalescent center in a Bremen home. After Mrs. Myers's sudden death, the Church of the Brethren took over but couldn't handle the financial burden. The people of German Township and surrounding areas raised money, bought the home, incorporated the Community Hospital of German Township as a not-for-profit community hospital, and got it licensed by the state. The legislature authorized a small tax to help fund its operation.

Bremen needed a hospital. The community and surrounding area are twenty to thirty-five miles from Plymouth, Rochester, South Bend, Mishawaka, Elkhart, Warsaw, La Porte, and Goshen, where there are hospitals. Accidents often occur on the heavily traveled roads that go through or near Bremen. Amish families in slow-moving buggies are vulnerable and can't make good time going to a hospital. Farm and factory accidents are numerous.

The State Board of Health once threatened to close the hospital because it was small. The community turned out en masse for a hearing, and the board's representatives learned in no uncertain terms that Bremen needed and wanted its hospital. Even the Amish turned out. The hospital subsequently was relicensed.

The hospital then had about fifteen beds. It was remodeled and expanded to twenty-three beds in 1958. In 1977 citizens dipped into their pockets to create a modern hospital with twenty-eight beds. The hospital was the first with OB convalescent rooms next to a nursery equipped with delivery drawers so that mothers can hold and feed their babies when they wish. In the early eighties, the community raised $800,000 to add the latest diagnostic and treatment equipment. In 1990 the hospital added an emergency department, more than doubled outpatient capacity, and added radiology, physical therapy, and cardiac rehabilitation.

South Bend and Mishawaka specialists of all types now spend a day a week in Bremen seeing patients. There are seven physicians, a long way from May 31, 1946, when Doctor Cripe and I began practicing as the new—and only—doctors in town.

Supply and demand remains the answer to attracting doctors to small towns. If U.S.-trained doctors prefer larger communities with more sophisticated hospitals and greater opportunity to specialization, then doctors trained outside the country have splendid opportunities as general practitioners in areas with unmet needs. Small towns advertise, build doctor's offices, and offer amenities because they understand the fierce competition for doctors. They want their own physicians. They should have them.

Closed-circuit television and other types of remote consultation with specialists may mean more rural areas without doctors in the future. Bremen would have faced that danger if its physicians and townspeople had lacked foresight. Luckily as a rapidly growing bedroom community, Bremen's increasing need for medical services will support the hospital and hold good physicians. Other towns may not be as fortunate.

On a personal level, our family found Bremen to be the "good town" promised by the signs at the town limits. Its good schools, parks, and churches reflect the values of its thrifty, honest people, many of whom are of German descent.

In a small-town practice, finding time for family is a difficult challenge for which there is no medical school preparation. Beth did most of the child-rearing. Without ever complaining, she was our children's mother, part-time father, chauffeur, disciplinarian, and counselor. Most of the responsibility for school activities fell to her.

As much as possible for a busy country doctor, I tried to help. I cooked breakfast on Sunday mornings so that Beth could get the kids off to Sunday school. I did the yard work. In winter, I shoveled our walks. Our house was on a corner lot, so there was twice as much sidewalk to clear. I also cleared sidewalks for an elderly couple living next door.

We tried to do things as a family. An example was our annual trip to a tree farm to cut a Christmas tree. Even when it was snowing and cold, the kids enjoyed it. We had room to display a large tree, and our children thought "bigger was better." Once they spied the one they wanted and we began cutting it, they learned that bigger wasn't necessarily easier. However, everyone took a turn with the saw.

I spent less time with my children than I wanted, but I have wonderful memories from their earlier days. They might prefer that I remain silent about their occasional mischief, but some of the things they did are fun to talk about now.

In my years of practice, real vacations were rare. The only way a physician can relax is to get out of town. That's never easy. Arrangements must be made for another doctor to take calls, and OB patients due to deliver must be told which doctor is substituting. Our most memorable vacations were to Indiana, Michigan, Wisconsin, and the Canadian lakes.

This period—when I was practicing and Beth and I were rearing our family—was fulfilling and rewarding both personally and professionally. I've always said that work isn't work if you enjoy what you're doing. I was busy doing what I enjoyed. My only regret is that my practice, politics, and government kept me from spending more time with my children. I now realize that Beth carried a far greater share of the load of rearing our family than she should have. I supplied the wherewithal, but she had the most important task.

This also was a challenging period. I became accustomed to long hours, lost sleep, and missed meals. I learned to remain calm and unflustered and to be patient with and tolerant of others. I learned when to be tactful and when to be stern and decisive.

In short, as a doctor, father, and neighbor, I learned a great deal that would serve me well in public life.

Excerpts from chapter 5, Doc: Memories from a Life in Public Service *by Otis R. Bowen, MD, with William Du Bois Jr., copyright 2000, Otis R. Bowen, MD, Indiana University Press (2000), reprinted with permission of IU Press.*

Editor's Note: My favorite story about Doctor Bowen takes place at the September 2005 dedication of the Historic Family Doctor's Office exhibition at the Indiana Medical History Museum in Indianapolis. Bowen and I were the speakers for the ceremony and we were sitting in the front of the room chatting as the audience gathered and found their seats in the museum's large, beautiful medical amphitheater. As we sat Bowen asked me, "See that person over there? I can't remember his name."

I told him the name.

"And that fellow over there? His name escapes me."

I replied with his name.

"Oh, yes of course!" he responded. "And one more, that guy in the blue sport coat?"

I once again told him this person's name.

"Thanks, Richard." Bowen said softly.

After Bowen delivered his keynote address and the dedication proceedings were completed, a throng of people came down to the front to greet him. Every one of those individuals remarked to me how pleased and impressed they were that Bowen could remember their names after so many years.

Even at nearly ninety years old, Otis Bowen was ever the politician!

3

Three Generations of Family Docs

Frank Beardsley, MD

I never thought of any career other than medicine. My dad was a doctor, and I always loved what he did. He would take me on house calls and to the hospital. My father attended medical school in Chicago, and then went to Minnesota, where he met my mother and married her. He came back to Champaign, Illinois, and established a practice. He did the first C-section ever done there. Doctor Bergen here in Frankfort, Indiana, urged him to come back, so he came back here in 1921. He was a general practitioner at a time when they really did everything. He did all kinds of surgery, gave anesthesia, delivered babies, all kinds of orthopedics, the whole nine yards. In those days, doing all that was not at all unusual.

We were going to practice together, but he had a heart attack and died in May of that year. I was planning to come back to town in June. I really loved him. My dad and I were really close. The day he died, I think, was the saddest day of my life. It was so sudden.

I started my practice on my thirtieth birthday in 1955. Dad had an X-ray machine in his office and a room full of prescription medications he would give to patients. He had a 5x7 card for each family. On one

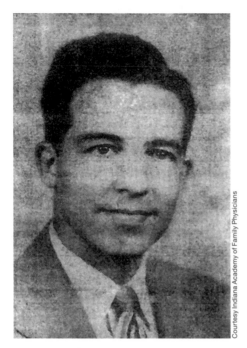

Courtesy Indiana Academy of Family Physicians

Frank Beardsley

side was the financial record, and the other side was the medical history. So, that's what I started with. After about two to three months, people came in to talk about their problems, and I had no idea what they were talking about. I decided that I would have to have a more complete record, so I started with regular-sized paper and files. Everything was handwritten, of course.

When I started, I expect I worked fourteen-hour days for probably the first fifteen to sixteen years. For the next ten years, I probably still put in twelve hours a day. Then, I gave up anesthesia and obstetrics and started working less. Since I had open-heart surgery, I have cut down to about twenty hours a week.

I borrowed $1,500 from the bank for cash flow when I started. After six months, I had $500 of bills on my desk and no money to pay them. I said to my father-in-law, "I didn't know what to do. I couldn't have been working any harder. I was extremely busy from the day I took over his practice, and I never slowed down." He told me that I would have to raise my fees. I was charging two dollars for an office call and a dollar for medicines, so patients walked out of my office with a bill of three dollars for complete care. So, I raised my prices to three dollars for an office call. In about two to three years, I finally had my head above water. I wasn't rich, but I wasn't sinking either. I think I charged five dollars for a house call at that time. I made a lot of house calls.

There was a flu epidemic one year, and I made seventeen house calls one day. I usually made a few every day. I gave anesthetics, delivered probably seventy-five babies a year, had a very active office practice, and made hospital rounds on my patients. I usually didn't stop for lunch. My nurses would leave at 6:00 p.m., and I usually still had three to four patients yet to see. I would typically leave the office somewhere between 7:00 p.m. or 8:00 p.m. and still had two to three house calls to make. I'd get home at 9:00 p.m. lots of times and my kids were already in bed. There was an emergency room at that time, but it wasn't staffed. So, if somebody called in the middle of the night with chest pain, I couldn't say "go to the ER" or "this is nothing." I had to get up and go see the patient. I would guess that I made about five calls during the week between midnight and 5:00 a.m.

I still make a few house calls today, as I always have. But I think because emergency rooms have become so active, and urgent care centers have popped up all over, there is not as much of a need for house calls. But there is another reason why I still don't make house calls as much as I used to. When I started, we had more of an unscientific approach in medicine, and we didn't have a whole lot of things to work with or to offer patients. We could do about as well in the home as we could in the office. But now we have so many more things to work with in our offices and our hospitals that it doesn't make sense to see a lot of illnesses in the home any more.

The rewards of the job have changed some over the years. When I started, I think the rewards were the love and respect we had for our patients, and the love and respect our patients had for us. There was a loyalty we had for each other. Although these things are still present, I don't think they are present to the same extent that they were. I practiced thirty-six years, and my practice had so much loyalty. Most of my patients were like family. I run into patients all the time and they say something like, "You delivered me!" I still like to hear that kind of stuff.

Now there are so many malpractice suits. All people make mistakes, including doctors, no matter how smart you are or anything. Litigation was not at all like it is today. People accepted the fact that everything might not turn out exactly as expected. They were more accepting.

I think I've learned an awful lot about human nature in this profession. Believe it or not, the most common problems we see probably have their root in anxieties and stress. Far and away, the most common fundamental thing that brings most people to the doctor has to do with their emotions.

When I started practicing medicine, one thing that was really great was that you were your own boss, and you did what you wanted to do. You did simply what you thought was right. Now you have so many people looking over your shoulder at everything you do. I enjoy my work very much. But in the last ten years, there have been lots of changes that I don't like. I think if I started practice today, I don't think I would be happy at all. There are so many rules and regulations today. I don't think it's as much fun.

Money has become a bigger factor in medicine in the last decade. I remember my father always told me that if I wanted to get rich, I was going into the wrong profession. He said, "You will make decent money, you will have a roof over your head, all the food you need, and a good life. But you will never be wealthy." I think that was accurate. I think today, some specialists are in it more for the money than for the doctoring.

When I started practicing, there were a lot of general practitioners, and there were also some surgeons, internists, and orthopedic surgeons, and OB/GYNs. They weren't overspecialized, and they didn't overcharge. It was a nice balance. Then all of a sudden we've got a specialist for anything and everything, and they can make a million dollars a year or more. There are an awful lot of guys who are more interested in the big bucks. That has made medicine more of a business than a service. There are too many people who have gone that way. Primary care physicians will make less money than any other group of doctors, but in many ways they will provide a better service. I'm afraid many specialists are just looking at one organ and not knowing or caring about anything else about the patient. The family practitioner is holistic.

But years ago, the general practitioner was not considered a specialist. Today, there is a specialty called family medicine. It requires a three-year residency just like every other specialty, and it requires a board exam with retesting at least every seven years. There was a grandfather clause when the American Board of Family Practice originated, and if you didn't complete a residency but you kept up with postgraduate work since medical school, you could take the Boards. I did and passed. The only way you can sit for your Boards today is after a three-year residency. The general public doesn't realize that family practice is a specialty. There is a lack of respect for family practitioners, and it is not justified.

I have also always been a member of the American Academy of Family Physicians, and they have always required at least 150 hours of Continuing Medical Education every three years. I have done that ever since I got out of medical school. I think family practice was the biggest proponent of the idea of CME, and other specialties have followed suit.

Family doctors are probably doing more for wellness now than they ever have. The most common cause of death in America today is heart disease. We have been learning the things we need to know about cholesterol to prevent heart attacks. Because of what we learned from the compilation of the results of many studies, we know that for every percentage point we lower the cholesterol, we can lower heart disease by 2 percent. So, we know that if we can get Americans on a low-cholesterol diet, we can greatly reduce the number of deaths from heart disease. I predict that in twenty years, by the time the grocery stores and restaurants get more cholesterol minded, and we do not have a lot of cholesterol in our diets, we will likely eliminate 90 percent of heart disease in America.

Speaking of preventive medicine or the lack of it, many doctors smoked when I went into practice. I would get a call, and on the way to the call I would have a cigarette. On the way back I would have a cigarette. When the alarm went off in the morning, I would have a cigarette. Then I would smoke a cigarette after breakfast. I'd have a cigarette on my way to the hospital, and a lot of times I'd smoke a half pack of cigarettes before my first surgery. Then, after surgery, I'd go into the doctors' room and have a cigarette. I had ashtrays on my desk, and I blew smoke in everybody's face all the time. I smoked about three packs a day for the first year and a half that I practiced medicine. We just didn't know the real dangers of smoking back then. I quit cold turkey from three packs a day. I haven't smoked for fifty years.

In my era medicine was a rather "unscientific science." It was a science, but it wasn't as exacting as it is today. Now with all the newer technologies, facilities, and medicines available, doctors are much more precise and safer in their work. It's not that we were sloppy in our day; we just didn't have the tools to work with.

Let me give you some examples of what I'm talking about: When we delivered a baby, there were three people in the room—the patient, a nurse who gave ether anesthetic, and the doctor. One of the worst scenarios that I remember was at three in the morning. A gal was bleeding like a stuck pig. There was no blood bank, of course. We called the lab technician who got dressed and came in and typed and cross matched the patient's blood. She was A positive, so she went down to look in her book for people who have signed up to donate blood. She called them in the middle of the night, and they came to the hospital. When they arrived, I broke scrub and went down and drew the blood from the volunteers. Then she had to type and cross match that blood, and only then could I finally give this woman the blood she desperately needed.

So, from the time that the gal started bleeding like hell, it was two to three hours before we had blood to give her. That was scary. Her husband was like a prisoner. He could not come near either the baby or his wife. The baby is born and whisked off to the nursery, and the mother is going down the tubes. We finally got her stable and moved her into a room. Only then could he see the mother. Then he could also go see the baby but only through the glass of the nursery. There was no closeness available for the families there at all.

By the time I quit obstetrics, there was a new obstetrical unit in the hospital with the rooms where the whole family could be there during labor. When it came time for the delivery, she stayed in the same bed and delivered right there. People could stay in the room during delivery, and they could all hold the baby immediately. What a difference between being a prisoner to being involved as much as you want to be. That is the way it should be. One of the big stumbling blocks back then was the risk of infection.

Let me also tell you about Doctor Compton and my father who decided to practice together. They had a surgery room in their office, and they did tonsillectomies there. The next room to that was a private office with a cot. They would give the anesthesia for each other for the tonsillectomies. As soon as they were through, they would put the child in the back room on the cot, and when they woke up they could go home.

It wasn't that much better when I started. My associate did the tonsillectomies, and he was fast. I would give the anesthesia. He had a long silver tongue blade with a hole in the end and a knife that would go through that hole. He would get the tonsil through there and have it cut out before you knew it. Then he would remove the adenoids in under a minute with another instrument. We would then start sucking the blood out to see where the bleeders were. He would clamp and suture the bleeder, and then he would watch it for three to four minutes. When there was no more bleeding, it was done. From the time he started to the time he was finished was about ten minutes.

There was no recovery room, so you picked up the child and put him on the cot in the room and called mother in. Here was the child vomiting blood and blue half the time. What a horrible sight. Now, of course, they go to the recovery room, and they use different anesthetics and medications to control vomiting. By the time they get back to the parents, they look pretty normal. It was really barbaric back then. I don't know how they all lived. I never had a tonsil death. Probably should have. I do remember a child in town of another doctor who died on the table. That was a tragedy. Thankfully, we've come a long way since those times.

I have had a wonderful rewarding career. But the one thing that I really hated about the practice of medicine was that I couldn't do justice to both medicine and my family at the same time. Maryann raised the kids and did a great job. My oldest son is a family physician at Franciscan Saint Francis Health in Beech Grove, just outside of Indi-anapolis. He started both a practice and teaching at the family practice residency in 1981. He has done that every day of his career since then. He is very bright and very dedicated. I'm proud of him. He is the best doctor that I have ever known.

Taken from the transcript of Doctor Beardsley's interview.

4

The Son of a Family Doctor

Nick Frank Hrisomalos, MD

Frank Hrisomalos, MD, was born on April Fools' Day, 1929. He grew up as the only child of two Greek immigrants and graduated from Bloomington High School in Bloomington, Indiana, in 1946. He graduated with a pharmacy degree from Purdue University in 1951 before attaining his undergraduate degree from Indiana University in 1952. Hrisomalos graduated from the IU School of Medicine in 1956. After graduation, he moved to Bloomington and started his solo private practice. He is currently the longest practicing physician in Monroe County, Indiana.

"You kids want a Tin Roof?"

It was Saturday night, around 10:00 p.m. We were in the kitchen of one of my dad's patients while he was in the other room, doing a house call.

"Or maybe a banana split?"

My dad would always take us with him on house calls if we were home, especially if he hadn't seen us for a while. We loved it. It was fun to visit the patients and see their appreciation for medical care and personal attention. The side benefits were pretty good too!

I remember one time a yellow cab pulled up in our front driveway, the driver came to the door and rang the doorbell. The smell of a hot freshly cooked homemade pizza drifted through the house as we read the note scribbled on top of it—a thank you gift from a patient. To our surprise, my dad swiftly took the object of our desire and deposited it directly into the garbage can! Asking why, he told us about the bag of human hair the same patient had just sent him—a bag that had a note with it asking him to send the contents for toxicology and for arsenic, as the patient felt her husband was trying to poison her! The family practitioner has to deal with all varieties of patients and problems, the mental and the physical. And sometimes you just have to go hungry. I suppose some of those side benefits were better than others!

My dad, Frank Hrisomalos, MD, was born the son of two Greek immigrants. When he was born, the physician asked my grandmother "What is his name for the birth certificate?" My grandmother said "Theophanis"—after a second he responded, "That just won't do; we'll just call him Frank" (after himself!). After he finished college at Indiana University, he completed a pharmacy degree at Purdue and then went

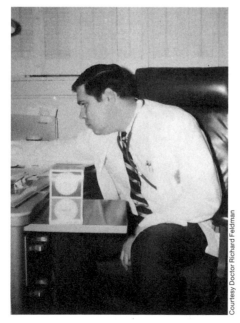

to medical school at IU in Indianapolis. He returned to Bloomington with a wife and a couple of kids and started an idyllic practice. "Doctor Frank," as everyone called him, could walk from his house, past the family restaurant, to his office that was just a few blocks down the street. He could easily walk to many of his patients' homes and walk or drive to the hospital for rounds.

He delivered babies and even went to Nashville,

Frank Hrisomalos

Courtesy Doctor Richard Feldman

Indiana, to perform anesthesia. Amazingly, thirty years after my father was born, he had to deliver his own daughter when the obstetrician could not be found! He was the epitome of the all-encompassing family physician. My dad loved his work, and his patients adored him and trusted him. Through his practice, his life was woven into the tapestry of all his patients' lives.

I don't sleep much, to this day. Just not used to it. Growing up, we would hear the phone ring all night. Oftentimes, we'd then hear dad closing the front door, starting up the car, and leaving for a delivery, emergency, or something like that. In the early morning, we'd go downstairs and see his black doctor's bag on the counter, always with a sinuous stethoscope tube peeking out. We would marvel at the pharmacopeia of bottles and pills inside along with the hammers, tongue blades, otoscope, and needles. It was like a magician's bag of tricks, intriguing and mysterious. Out of that bag, he could heal and help people, and the imagery was intriguing. My dad saved lives, gave meaning to lives, and made a difference. In return, he reaped the reward of an extremely fulfilling life.

My dad's bedroom was always littered with medical journals as far as one could see. They were ear marked and had pictures of organs and lists of indecipherable long medical names on their covers. He was always learning and educating himself, not just practicing what he learned in medical school. The family physician has so much to keep up on—the whole body is their specialty. What a perspective on life they compiled by virtue of their work—dealing with patients, their families, their births and their deaths—their struggles and their joys; the family doctor sees it all, and it's incredible.

Growing up as the son of a family physician was wonderful; we had a sunlit childhood. We were able to see the appreciation of patients, understand the hard work and discipline necessary to be successful, and learn how to think of others before yourself. My dad missed many a party or event because he felt a duty to his patients in distress. We could see the incredible enjoyment that he derived from his work and the good that came from it.

Playing golf on a Sunday afternoon, as we often did, we would see a golf cart racing towards us—cutting across the fairways, not following any type of protocol. It was the golf pro from the clubhouse—he had a message from the answering service. It was an emergency, in the day of no portable cell phones. We would hurriedly leave and head to the car where my dad had one of the first cell phones. It took up most of his trunk, and you had to call an operator to connect. At football games, they would page dad over the loudspeaker—maybe it was someone in labor ready to deliver!

We had a medical family. My mother helped us all deliver three baby teacup poodles in our bathroom using dental floss and rubber bands. She was always there to help when dad had to be gone. She helped all four of us children garner a taste for medicine by bringing home eyes, hearts and kidneys of cows from the slaughterhouse of a patient for us to dissect and learn. The family physician needs to have someone at home that is strong, self-sufficient, and willing to share their life with the practice.

Wiping the water out of my eye, I would reload my syringe and squirt a long stream of cold water at my brother. We had such fun toys, dad giving us all varieties and sizes of syringes to use as squirt guns. There were all sorts of penlights, and neat devices the pharmaceutical reps would leave.

We loved to go to the office, a converted house with white siding. We'd turn on the centrifuge and get it spinning until it "whirred." We would dunk urine dipsticks in all forms of liquids for fun, even the tiny five-cent bottles of Coca-Cola we'd get from the vending machine. It was fun to peer through the microscope at our fingerprints or lint we would find in the corner. Clacking the old Royal typewriter and running the ditto-spirit machine, with the aroma of the alcohol coming off the cool, smooth paper is still memorable. We took our fair share of candy Dum Dum lollypops from the big box on the shelf by the pediatrics rooms. The patients would always tell us hello. They'd say something about how much they appreciated our dad seeing them, especially if it was a Saturday or Sunday, which was common.

It was a privilege to grow up as the son of a family doctor. All the experiences we observed and participated in at an early age were remarkable. Seeing birth and death, despair and suffering, cures and satisfaction all made for an incredible childhood. I look up to the family physician as a true Renaissance person. They have a boundless work ethic, tremendous life perspective, and they give up their life for the benefit of others, producing such good in the world. I can see it from the outside and the inside, and I'm very proud of it.

I work on a postage stamp. My upbringing garnered a love of medicine and yearning to help people, and I elected to become a physician myself, specializing in the eye. More specifically, as an ophthalmologist, I specialize on the small, thin lining of the interior of the eye—the retina. The internally rewarding act of taking care of people was contagious in my family. My brother became a physician, my two sisters dentists, and my mother a social worker. Being a member of a family doctor's family gave all of us the urge to follow and help the human body and the soul lying within. A family physician must approach the body as a whole and appreciate how each piece is connected and works together. I am amazed at their ability to methodically piece apart these complicated interrelations as my specialty is entirely the opposite, focusing only on one small area of the body. As I peer into the depths of an eye, through the aperture of the pupil, I see the big picture emerge. The family doc looks at the whole person and tries to decipher oftentimes small problematic dysfunctions, using their expertise, experience, and the art of medicine. Importantly, medicine as we know it could not exist without these distinct yet complementary focuses.

The monstrous *Physicians' Desk Reference* (*PDR* as many call it) is now a dusty bookend in my dad's office. Things have changed. Information on drug interactions is a click away and anyone can get a hold of you on your pocket cell in a second. Payment by pizza is definitely declining. Although it's easier to keep up with current treatment and the stacks upon stacks of printed journals aren't as necessary, I think it's harder to keep up because of the voluminous amount of material and the pace of change. One thing hasn't changed, however; there are still only twenty-four hours in a day. The lifestyle and nostalgia of the Mayberry RFD physician is well on its way to the Star Trek version, and the family doctor is adapting amazingly well.

When I call and ask for medical clearance of a complicated, sick patient for their eye surgery or call about the need to treat diabetes, an infection, or another problem discovered through a retina exam, the family doc dutifully says, "No problem, we will get it done." Their willingness to embrace the patient as a whole and take responsibility for coordinating specialty care is admirable.

My dad is eighty-two years old and still works seven days a week. Can't get the drive out of him. It's spread to my children, one a physician and one soon to graduate medical school. My wife, similar to my mother, irreplaceably ties our medically focused family together. The wheel keeps turning.

5

Patients Are People

Eugene Gillum, MD

Prior to World War II, 80 percent of doctors did general practice and 20 percent were specialists. These guys went into the service, many for four to five years away from their practices. Some were in combat, but others were doing draft exams, tropical medicine, or in the South Pacific someplace treating malaria. When they got back from the war, they found what they did in the service was important, but it had no relationship to what they had done in their practice. There were tremendous changes in medicine taking place. There were changes in anesthesia, antibiotics (penicillin and sulfa), blood transfusions, and the treatment of shock to name a few. Many of these advancements were developed during the war.

These fellows came back to their hometowns, and the world had jumped a couple of steps ahead of them. There was an effort to do something to help physicians get updated to all of the scientific changes that occurred while they were away during the war. One result was the creation of the American Academy of General Practice. The Academy required that in order to belong to the organization, you had to do an average of fifty hours of postgraduate education each year. It saw the value of having some kind of managed continuing medical education specific for its type of medicine.

General practitioners also began to realize that there were certain things that set them apart from just the science of medicine. Two-thirds of what you do as a family doctor is science and the other third of it is the human side of medicine—understanding and knowing the patient as a person. Specialists just don't have the focus on the person. It's just different when you are the person of first contact. It's a natural part of being a primary care physician.

That's when the name of the organization changed to the American Academy of Family Physicians. We work in the context of the family. Part of the approach is appreciating the various influences at work in a patient's life. Part of it is genetic, part behavioral, part environmental, part economic, and part religious, political, and cultural. All these things affect a person's behavior; it affects who you marry, where you educate your children, and the prejudices you pass on to your family, etc. So, if you are going to do family practice well, you need to know something about the patient as a person and the influences of the family on that person. It boils down to this: Are you treating a disease or are you treating a person? Too often, specialists focus on the disease and the patient is secondary. Family docs treat the person who has a disease.

People are not diseases and they are not just numbers. When a patient comes to see you, you shut the door of the exam room. It's you and the patient on one side of the door. You shut the world out. You deal with the problem on a one-on-one personal basis then and there. Period.

Physicians have to deal with life and death. They have to learn in some way how to deal with death on a personal level. When a patient dies, it is always difficult. It affects you profoundly. It is certainly true in family practice because you know your patients so well over so many years.

I had a good friend who was in practice a little bit north of here. He loved to gamble and played poker on Saturday night. He was a football player in high school and on the golf team in college. He played everything to win. His life was being number one, period.

When you have somebody who is eighty-five years old and dying of pneumonia, you're not in a winning situation. You could be the Mayo Clinic and that patient is still going to die. What's that have to do with a doctor who is a born winner? He picked a specialty that didn't require him to deal with losing. Losing a patient was an insult, and it hurt him. He couldn't face death. He couldn't handle not being able to do anything about it. Physicians have to learn how to deal with death. I don't know exactly how you learn it; you might rely on your religion, but you really learn through experiencing it. It's the most difficult part of being a doctor.

I don't know of anything in this world that is more humbling than delivering a baby. There's no other thrill, nothing you will ever do for that family that is equivalent of presenting them with a healthy baby. Everything in life revolves around that. But delivering babies also teaches you that you can't solve all medical problems, and sometimes you lose. Without that experience, a medical student's education is lacking.

Sometimes I think it should be a requirement of all medical students to deliver fifty babies before graduation. I think someone who is going to call himself a physician ought to have that experience. If you do fifty deliveries, you're going to run into at least one case that bites you. You'll face a potentially life-threatening situation for either the mother or the baby.

My point is that I don't think someone ought to graduate medical school without ever having to face life and death. They need to appreciate the fragility of life.

Taken from the transcript of Doctor Gillum's interview.

6

Times Are Changing

Ray Nicholson, MD

My patients always came first. When I came into medicine there was a horrible doctor shortage. When 5:00 a.m. came, and someone thought their kid had pneumonia, there was nobody in the ER to see the child. And there were no urgent care centers to go to. So, either kids got nothing or you saw them. Most of my generation was just used to seeing people when they needed to be seen. That was always my attitude. It's different today; attitudes are changing.

I've been in practice for forty-eight years now. I have taught medical students my whole career, and I was a family medicine residency program director for twenty-eight years. I've never been "dumped on" in my life. I hear residents at rounds every day say, "Oh, they dumped on me again last night."

You see, it's all about the attitude. Maybe the "dump" came from a cardiologist who felt like the patient needed a good generalist to see him. Maybe the patient had a heart problem, but he also had diabetes and hypertension and some other things. Why would I think that that referral was a dump? The residents I teach sure do, though. They are learning not to say those things around me, because I have no sympathy for them.

In forty-eight years of practice, I only sent two people to collections. I think I probably do have a different attitude than many younger doctors. I never, ever allowed the nurse to tell me if a patient owed me money. When I saw the patient, if they owed me ten dollars or a thousand dollars, it didn't make any difference. I did not want to know that because I was fearful that my thinking would be influenced. The important thing was always the care of the patient.

The other thing is that I think we are losing the basics of good clinical diagnostic skills. Good diagnosticians really talk to the patient. They examine patients carefully. One day, the residents were telling me about a guy they thought had a subarachnoid (brain) hemorrhage. I asked what the CT showed, and they said it was normal. Only very rarely will the scan be normal in a hemorrhage. I said, "You've probably got the wrong diagnosis."

They said they had tried to do a spinal tap three times the night before, but they weren't able to get it. I said, "If you are right, we need to do a spinal tap."

So, I went down to talk to the patient before anyone else got into the room. I just listened to him and asked him if he had been having any personal problems or work problems. He said, "Nobody likes me at work. Everybody hates me but my boss. He thinks I hung the moon. But I got fired yesterday." I asked him what time of day it happened, and he said, "About 4:00." I asked him when the headache started, and he said, "4:10."

Obviously the residents were shocked and wanted to know how I got that out of him. I said, "Well for starters, you have to sit down and talk to the patient." In the long run, that may have taken a little more of my time, but can you imagine how much money we saved on his medical bill.

The number one complaint from patients about our residents, or other physicians for that matter, is that "he doesn't listen to me." I could never work for an HMO where you are expected to see a patient every ten minutes. I need to take the time to listen to what the patient has to say, their issues, and their concerns. It's an important part of taking

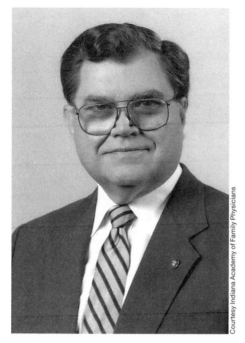

Courtesy Indiana Academy of Family Physicians

Ray Nicholson

good care of people and part of being a good doctor.

Physicians are so dependent on high technology that they are losing their history-taking and physical exam skills. They are less reliant on those things today. They think talking to the patient and performing a good physical exam is secondary. Once, one of the residents and I were looking at an MRI and a CT on a patient that he had seen, and I hadn't seen yet. The resident said, "I'm not sure what's wrong. I guess I'll go up and take a history and physical." That's the way most medicine is today. They've got it backwards.

Many physicians, especially medical educators, are also afraid that we are creating a new generation of doctors with a "shift attitude." That starts in residency training with the new duty hour restrictions that residency programs have to strictly follow. A resident can only work so long, and then they must go home to rest or sleep. When a resident works on call all night, he or she must not be present at the hospital for nearly the entire next day. If the residency violates these rules, it can lose its accreditation.

No one thinks residents should work to exhaustion or be abused, but these young physicians-in-training are missing out on a lot of valuable clinical experiences and medical education. Working long hours in residency training has historically been the norm, just as working long hours in practice was the customary situation as well.

I had a set of twins getting ready to deliver, and the resident called me at 4:30 in the afternoon and said the woman was moving along, and it wouldn't be long. So, I told the resident to hang around, and I'd let him deliver one. So, they called me at 5:05 p.m. that she was crowning. I couldn't find him and went on over to deliver the babies. The next day I saw him and said, "I hate that you missed the delivery last night, I was going to let you deliver the twins with my assistance." He said, "Too bad they didn't come before 5:00 before it was time for me to go home." Now, in my day, interns would stay up until 4:00 a.m. to deliver twins. I was shocked.

Just a couple of years ago, we were standing in surgery and the resident said, "Oh, it's 12:30. Time to go to lunch." He took off his gloves and went to lunch. I was about to say something to the surgeon and he said, "Let the son-of-a-bitch go."

I've had a wonderful career. Although in some respects, I think things are not headed in the best direction, in many ways the golden age of medicine is actually ahead of us. The technological and other advances in medicine are endless.

I've been running the muscular dystrophy clinic for fifteen years. I think in the next five years there will be blood tests for DNA, and we will be able to specifically say what type of muscular dystrophy it is and have gene therapy for that. I think there is a bright future ahead through DNA testing and gene therapy, and we will be able to cure cancer in the not-so-distant future.

If you look at when I started in practice, we had not a single diuretic available. We had digitalis, but no beta blockers, calcium channel blockers, ACE inhibitors, nothing. We only had Thorazine and Phenobarbital for psychiatric issues. We were limited to Dilantin and Phenobarbital for seizures. We had three antibiotics. We had only standard X-rays—no CTs or MRIs. We couldn't measure thyroid and other physiologic parameters as we can today. Some people don't really get the point. They almost laugh at what we did. But it worked. People were cured. We did things that were innovative for the time that people laugh at today. But we saved lives. We used what we had available to us. We were very sincere in what we did.

Taken from the transcript of Doctor Nicholson's interview.

7

Looking Back and Looking Forward

Charles Rau, MD

Charles Rau, MD, was born January 29, 1934. He attended Indiana University for his undergraduate degree, which he received in anatomy and physiology in 1955. He graduated from the IU School of Medicine in 1958. Rau then completed an internship at Methodist Hospital in Gary, Indiana.

Rau began practicing in 1959, working in a two-physician group at Columbus Regional Hospital. His practice includes obstetrics and inpatient hospital work. One of Rau's notable accomplishments is that he has directed three free clinics for underprivileged people since 1971. He continues to practice medicine today.

My Medical Training

In most of my classes at Indiana University School of Medicine, I sat near Ben Ranck because of alphabetical seating. He and I ended up working at Community Hospital in Indianapolis for part of our training. Even though we were still medical students, we took care of all the emergencies, delivered the babies, and started all the IVs. I probably delivered 200 babies at Community Hospital. By the time we got out of med school we were really seasoned clinicians, and then he and I moved on to Methodist Hospital in Gary for our internships.

When Ben and I completed our internships, we decided to become partners and opened an office together. That was in 1959, and medical partnerships were unheard of in Indiana in those days. We selected Columbus as a location. We were the first doctors to open an office there in ten years.

Our original office space was a remodeled grocery store, and the adjacent space in the building was occupied by a radio repair shop. A few years later, still in the days before transistor radios, the radio shop put up a sign that read, "Tubes Tested Free." That was long before it was professionally acceptable for physicians to advertise, and another family doctor in town (who had a reputation as a jokester) moved the "Tubes Tested Free" sign from the shop to our entry door. Then he photographed the sign, took the picture to the medical society, and lodged a complaint against us for advertising.

The Practice when I Began

Our practice really boomed, right from the start. Ben and I had training that the other docs didn't have, and that ten-year gap helped us to outshine our competitors. Most of the docs who were practicing in Columbus when we arrived had been trained during World War II in hurry-up medical school programs, and they lacked knowledge of newer developments. For example, this was early in the era of antibiotic therapy, and a lot of those doctors didn't grasp the fact that when you treated a streptococcal infection with penicillin, you had to prescribe it for ten days. They were prescribing penicillin for three or four days.

Also, at that time there was virtually no postgraduate education. Once doctors started practicing, they didn't go back for more formal learning. But the American Academy of Family Physicians and the Indiana Academy were new organizations. We joined and benefited from the continuing education programs they required for membership. It was a new concept, and if I hadn't done that, I don't know where I would be today.

Training is a good thing, but as with most things, luck helps. In

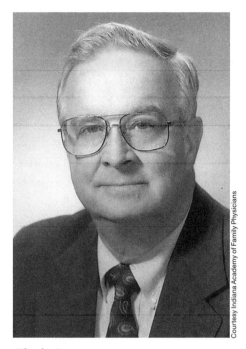

Courtesy Indiana Academy of Family Physicians

Charles Rau

1967 I was in the local Chrysler dealer's garage when one of the mechanics just keeled over and started turning blue. The modern approach to resuscitating people had just come out, and I had barely been taught this newfangled thing of chest pumping and mouth breathing. I started pumping his chest, and soon the ambulance arrived. At the hospital, they shocked him four or five times, his heart stabilized, and he was able to go home. I saved his life, but at the time I forgot that, in addition to pumping his chest, I was supposed to breathe for him.

Now, in the last year or two, it has come out that the breathing part is not necessary; all you need to do is pump the chest. I was inadvertently ahead of my time, as it turns out.

House Calls, Then and Now

In the early days, doctors made a lot of house calls. We took phone calls at home, and we didn't have a hospital operator between us and the patients at night. If we were out, our wives had to stay home and answer the phone. That arrangement was very confining, but that was the kind of devotion doctors and their families gave to their patients.

House calls these days, though, make a lot less sense. You need to remember that back then, there was about as much technology in the patient's house as there was in an emergency room. At that time, you had to work more on the basis of clinical impressions than diagnostic technology. Nowadays, because of the technology that can be applied in the emergency room, we do not, for instance, even let a chest pain come into our office. We direct them to the emergency room because you've got to make a diagnosis quickly. In a hospital, they can be worked into the cath lab, a stent can be put in, and they go home the next day.

Even when I started practice, we were selective about house calls and made them only if it was difficult for the patient to get to the office or if they were in too much pain. We never had to make house calls to drum up business. I still make a house call now and then, but it's pretty rare. House calls impress patients, but because of a lack of available technology there, they are generally a poor idea.

The "Good Old Days" Were Not Really That Good

In the early days of my practice, the technology simply did not exist. I have heard it said that before World War II, all a doctor had was morphine, digitalis, and surgery. Back when I started, in 1959, we were not a whole lot better off. What we didn't know probably didn't bother us, but based on what I know now, I sure wouldn't want to go back. We thought we were pretty sharp, you know, but in a way we really were not because of the state of the art at that time.

But I will say that as time has passed, I've come to realize that you can never arrive because medicine is always changing. It's like trying to catch up with the horizon. You can't get comfortable and say, "I know it all now," like old docs used to do when I started practice. They had fallen into that because medicine had changed so little for so long.

So were those early years of my practice "The Good Old Days"? I may have thought they were then, but I don't think so now.

Preventive Medicine—The New Personal Approach to Medicine

One thing we did not do for patients when I began the practice was pay any attention to wellness; we only responded to them when they had a medical problem. Later, we began to pay some attention to preventive medicine, but an awful lot of what we did was still reactive; when a patient got sick, you treated them and maybe had to put them into the hospital.

My son, David, and I have had a medical practice together for some time now. In the early 1990s, he and I started hitting the preventive thing very hard, particularly controlling cholesterol and blood pressure. I know that today we have many patients who are really healthy because we treated them so intensively. For instance, in the month of April of this year, 2009, we did not have one patient in the hospital. Physicians used to wait until a patient crashed, but now we try to prevent the crash.

An important aspect of preventive medicine is making sure the patients follow instructions, taking the right medications at the right times, that sort of thing. And that is where, these days, the physician-patient relationship is so important in our practice. From what I read in the journals, most patients do not do what their doctors tell them— like take their pills—but with the relationship I have with my patients, when I tell them to do something, they generally do it. They trust me, and I believe they respect me. We've been together for so long.

Another reason they follow instructions, though, is our scheduling policy; no patient leaves our office without an appointment to come back. If they are really sick, they may have an appointment to come back in a week. Or the appointment is made up to six months before they return if they are relatively healthy. In that way, they know we're interested in them, and they know that we will follow up on what they have been doing. All this builds strong interpersonal relationships. This is why I like family practice rather than a specialty.

By controlling cholesterol and hypertension, most of my patients who are all old now, have gotten through the cardiovascular period of their lives. Now our eighty year olds are getting cancer. Their immune systems gradually age and they don't neutralize the cancer cells like they did. The big problem with cancer is that we cannot treat it preventively as well as we can with coronary artery disease. We've been working on vitamin D deficiency with our patients in the last year or two because if you are low on vitamin D, you double your chances of developing cancer because it influences the immune system.

Practicing preventive medicine can present problems, though. Back when Pap smears were brand new, it was not unusual in our office for a woman to come in with a medical problem and never have had a Pap smear in her life. In addition to treating those patients, we would routinely do a Pap smear. Well, it got back to us that one of the patients had complained to somebody. She called us "dirty doctors" because she had come in with a strep throat, and we did a Pap smear on her. But those Pap smears found a lot of cervical cancer that would have been missed otherwise.

Concentrating on wellness and preventive medicine is definitely the way to go. Our patients not only live longer now, they also have a better quality of life.

Role of Psychotherapy in Family Medicine

No antidepressants were available until the 1960s, just as there were no high-blood pressure medicines until 1973. I learned early on how to use psychopharmacology to treat depression. Since depression is either the first or second most frequently occurring disease, having some ability to deal with it helped a lot. When you save a patient who is about ready to throw in the towel and who has given up on life from their depression, they tend to give you the credit even though the medication is what did the job. As far as they are concerned, it is a miracle.

It was largely in the area of dealing with emotional problems that family physicians became the counselors and the go-to guys for the whole population. Their role with patients was very close to the role that religious ministers had played in the past. This is another area in which interpersonal relationships with patients is so very important. Pharmacology may have solved the problem, if the problem was a chemical one. But there is also the emotional background; something may have caused the depression, whether it was a family problem or something else, and you end up discussing that with them.

My Practice Today

I've been practicing for over fifty years, and I haven't taken on a new patient in fifteen years. My son, David, takes all the new ones. The patients I have now are seventy through 100 years old, and a lot of them have been with me through forty or fifty years. That kind of continuity of care can be a great advantage in treating patients, but it can also create problems. The physician is apt to ascribe a patient's problem to a condition he has previously treated that patient for. To me that is a great worry. A patient comes in with a symptom and you are apt to say to yourself, "Oh, that's Mrs. Jones's irritable bowel syndrome acting up again," and it is really cancer of the ovaries. That's particularly true of patients who complain a lot, and one of these days they show up when they really are sick.

I am still practicing at my age of seventy-five for two reasons. One is, these folks are my friends, and I have shepherded them along for so long. I am confident that our new approach since the early 1990s, preventive medicine, has made a great difference in the health of our patients. I really have a stable full of old folks now.

The other reason I am still practicing is because over the years I have accumulated a fair amount of knowledge, and I feel like it would be a tremendous waste for me to retire now. Financially, I could retire and my wife would like that. It's not that I lack hobbies. I have several hobbies—gardening, fishing, hunting, and I grow grapes and make wine from them—but I really enjoy coming down here. I'm only in my office for three days a week now, but I'm on full call.

A new challenge to family medicine is the arrival of hospitalists—physicians who take care of patients only in the hospital. We have them in our hospitals now. We need to find a way for family doctors to maintain continuity of care while their patients are in the hospital, and they need to get paid for it. This is a hot issue right now. Having the family physician involved in hospital care greatly adds to the overall quality of medical care.

Medicine and Community Involvement

Back in the 1970s the community became aware that there were children in Columbus who were not receiving proper medical treatment. We established a child-care clinic to deal with that problem, and I've been an active participant from the start. We saw kids from ages one to six years old. We were greatly underfunded, but yet we charged nothing. In the 1980s we broadened our treatment to include everyone, regardless of age, and we called it the Health Care and Referral Clinic.

Nurses in the public health department would see people and triage them. By that time, we were funded just a little better, but the community wasn't really on board yet. That project did some good, though, and then in the early 1990s the concept of Volunteers in Medicine came around. We jumped on that right away, then suddenly, the whole community became active and we were very generously funded. In addition, we get free medicine from pharmaceutical companies. We don't see people who have insurance, and they have to make less than the median income in Columbus to be eligible. They are the working poor.

The whole project rides on my medical license these days, and I sign the prescriptions for the medications that the drug companies give for free. This year we brought $2.7 million worth of free medicine into this community. It has just gradually moved up in amount every year. Eli Lilly looked us over and decided we were the poster kids for the whole country, because we did it right. Both primary care physicians and specialists in the community are involved.

I'm very proud of what I've been able to contribute to these community-health projects, and I consider that activity to be an integral part of my practice of medicine.

Giving back is important.

Taken from the transcript of Doctor Rau's interview.

8

Passing the Torch

Deborah Allen, MD

Lester D. Bibler, MD, is considered the father of family medicine in Indiana; he is also considered one of the founding fathers of the American Academy of Family Physicians.

Bibler was born in Findlay, Ohio, in 1902. His family moved to Muncie, Indiana, where he received his primary education. He then attended Butler University for two years. Transferring to Indiana University, he graduated from the IU School of Medicine in 1925.

Upon his return from six years of service as a commander in the U.S. Navy during World War II, be began a private practice in family medicine in Indianapolis. He had a large practice there for many years and is remembered as a model family physician and mentor to generations of family doctors.

Concerned about the "encroachment of specialty groups in hospital organizations leading to the limitation of privileges for the general practitioner," Bibler played a central role in organizing general practitioners on a national level, culminating in the formation of the American Academy of General Practice in 1947 (later becoming the American Academy of Family Physicians). He served on its first board of directors in 1948 and was elected as vice president in 1952. He was also active in the formation of the Indiana chapter and served as its first president.

Bibler was a charter Diplomat of the American Board of Family Practice in 1969. He died in 1984.

The only spot left in the doctor's dining area was next to an elderly gentleman. Where were all of the other medical students? I was finishing a surgery elective during my senior year, and the last thing I wanted was to be stuck next to an old geezer and have to talk to him during lunch. There were no other options, so I sat down.

He was pleasant and engaged in a very polite conversation with me. I noticed immediately he was wearing a very unusual tie tack. It looked like two people holding hands with a child in between them. I had never seen anything like that and knew it must mean something to him. It was well worn and obviously a favorite of his. I asked what the tie tack represented.

He looked up at me and started to beam. "That represents a family," he said. "I am a family doctor, and I like to remind myself of who I am." I told him that I was going into family practice and was hoping to get into a residency program in Indianapolis.

He immediately started taking off the pin. I was dumfounded. What was he doing? He proudly handed me the tie tack and said that I should wear it like he had. Wear it proudly and always remember that it is a privilege to be a family physician. I tried to give it back to him, but he would not hear of it. He got up and left the table with me staring at the odd piece of jewelry I had just inherited. Who was that man?

I asked around and none of the students knew who the gentleman was, but one of the older surgeons recognized him and told me that was "old Doc Bibler." I put the name away in my memory banks and the tie tack in my jewelry drawer.

It would be years before I would even think about the tie tack again. As a senior resident, I started to receive publications from the Society of Teachers of Family Medicine and recognized its logo immediately. There on the top of the first page was the same logo used as the basis for

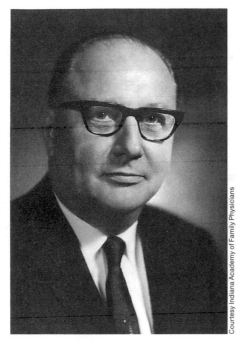

Lester D. Bibler

Courtesy Indiana Academy of Family Physicians

"my" tie tack! At least I knew where he got it from. He didn't tell me he had been a teacher. Who was that man?

I finished my residency in family practice at Methodist Hospital in Indianapolis in 1979 and stayed on to become a "Teacher of Family Medicine" myself. I served as the Associate Residency Director for seven years. During that time, I developed a much keener awareness of family medicine in Indiana. We were the largest specialty group of physicians in the state, but the Indiana University School of Medicine still did not require any medical student to learn about family medicine in the curriculum. Any exposure to family physicians was accomplished though groups of family doctors in the community who met regularly with interested students.

In my foolish naiveté, I left Methodist to become a faculty member in the IU Department of Family Medicine with the goal of getting family medicine in the curriculum of the medical school. Doctor Otis Bowen had just been asked by President Ronald Reagan to serve as the Secretary of Health and Human Services. He had been the Director of Medical Student Education in the Department of Family Medicine. I interviewed for his position and got the job.

Shortly after joining IU School of Medicine, I discovered that the Bibler family had started an endowment in the Department of Family Medicine. The funds have been, and continue to be used, to support a faculty member who contributes a large portion of their time to administration of the department. The faculty person who uses this endowment is known as the Lester Bibler Professor. This man had been committed enough to family medicine to give his own money to fund a permanent faculty position in the department.

I had been active in the Indiana Academy of Family Physicians, and I was in line to become president shortly after I changed jobs. At one IAFP meeting, I took some interest in looking at those who had previously been presidents and there at the very top of the list was Doctor Lester Bibler. Doctor Bibler had been the first president of the Indiana Academy of Family Physicians in 1948 (at that time called the Indiana Academy of General Practice). Jackie Schilling, the IAFP executive director, filled in some more information. I found out that he had been a member of the original group from the American Medical Association that started meeting to create the "specialty" of family practice in the early 1960s. She had several pictures of the group meeting at the AMA. There in the pictures sat a youthful and vigorous Lester Bibler fighting for the right for family practice to become a recognized specialty. I decided then and there that I was going to invite Doctor Bibler to my inauguration as president of the IAFP and tell him that I was the student he had so graciously given his STFM tie tack to so many years ago.

Doctor Bibler died two years before I was installed as the IAFP president. I never had the chance to tell him that he had indeed passed the symbol of his specialty on to a young student who eventually became the thirty-ninth president of the IAFP. I don't know if he even knew my name.

As so many things in life, "What goes round comes round." In 1989 I became Chair of the Department of Family Medicine and was responsible for the department's endowments. I received a call from the Development Office at the IU School of Medicine and David Bibler wanted to bring his ailing mother to the department and see what was being done with the Bibler endowment. I was thrilled to finally meet Vera Bibler and one of their sons. Vera was confined to a wheelchair and David wheeled her in to my office with the representative of the IU Foundation. After several minutes of formalities, she asked if I had known Lester. I told her that I had the pleasure of meeting him. She said, "If you knew him then you must have a story about him. Please tell me a story." I was near tears as I sat and told the Bibler family the story of the older family doctor and the young medical student and the official passing on of the tie tack. Vera Bibler beamed.

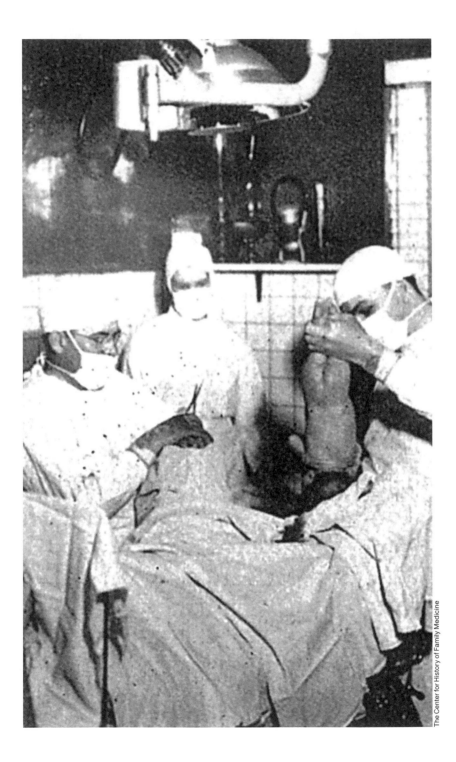

Part 2
Family Practice Stories

9

The Art of Using Placebos

Max Feldman, MD, was born in the Austro-Hungarian Empire in 1909. Immigrating to America in 1920, he spent the remainder of an impoverished childhood in New York City. He worked as a shipping clerk and attended night classes for two years at Brooklyn College, transferring to City College of New York as a full-time student and graduating in 1932.

Feldman returned to Europe for medical school, first attending the school in Konigsberg, Germany, for one year until Adolf Hitler came to power in 1933. Not feeling safe as a Jewish student in Germany, even as an American, he transferred to the University of Basil Medical School in Switzerland, graduating in 1937.

Returning to the United States, Feldman completed a one-year internship at Lincoln Hospital in New York City and a one-year internship at the U.S. Public Health Service Hospital on Staten Island. As a member of the U.S. Army Reserves, he joined the Civilian Conservation Corps as a medical officer in northern Wyoming for one year. He then activated and was sent to Fort Francis E. Warren in Cheyenne, Wyoming.

After assignments in Kansas and Missouri, Feldman was transferred to Tripler Army Hospital at Pearl Harbor in 1941 and served with distinction

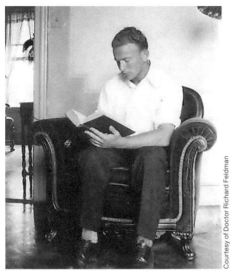

Max Feldman in Basil, Switzerland ca. 1933

Courtesy of Doctor Richard Feldman

as a young medical officer during the Japanese attack on December 7, 1941. He received additional assignments in the Pacific theater and in the United States.

Feldman was discharged from the military in 1946 and relocated his young family to South Bend, Indiana, where he was a family doctor in solo practice until he retired in 1983. His practice included hospital work, obstetrics, and some surgical procedures.

Feldman retired to Mountain View, California, and later to Seattle, Washington. He died in 2003.

The practice of medicine has changed in many ways over the years. Although it would be generally considered unethical nowadays, giving a patient a placebo was commonplace during the mid-twentieth century. Why were placebos more likely to be prescribed? It was certainly a time of greater paternalism in medicine. Doctors felt freer to utilize patient trust and longstanding doctor-patient relationships to improve their patients' lives, even if it meant being a bit deceptive. Certainly, we simply had fewer effective medicines available to treat many conditions. Regardless of the reasons, doctors were much freer to practice the "art of medicine." It surely must have made their day more fun.

The following story told to the author by his father, Doctor Max Feldman, would probably not occur today:

One day a middle-aged man came in to see my father at his office.

My father entered the room, and after they exchanged greetings my father asked, "What can I do for you today?"

"Doc, I've lost my nature."

"You lost your nature?" my dad asked in response.

"Yeah doc, it just doesn't seem to work anymore," replied the patient with a downcast look.

My father said that he had just the thing to help him. He left the room and returned with a small envelope full of pink aspirin and said: "Here is some medicine that will take care of your problem. Take one or two tablets about an hour before you plan to have sex. These pills are very strong. So, don't ever, ever, take more than two pills in one day! Do you understand? It's very important."

The man looked down at the envelope of pills as my father handed it to him. Then he looked wide-eyed up at my father and said, "Yes sir, Dr. Feldman, I won't ever take more than two. Thank you!"

A few weeks later the gentleman returned to my father's office for a minor illness. My father asked, "By the way, how did those pink pills I gave you work?"

The patient replied, "Doc, if they worked any better you would have to tie me to a tree!"

10

It's Time for Your Physical

Here is another example of the paternalism that existed during the golden era of family medicine. Doctors and their staff could just be more direct with their patients, and sometimes with patients who were not their patients.

This story was related to the author many years ago by his father, Max Feldman:

One day my father's receptionist noticed that one of his patients was late in coming in for his yearly physical. She pulled out his patient chart to call him. She thought she would extend a reminder to him about his physical and schedule his appointment. But there was no current phone number in the chart. So, she looked up the number in the phonebook and made the call. The patient's wife answered and scheduled his appointment with the receptionist and thanked her.

A week later, a very well-known golf pro from one of the local city courses arrived at the office. Now, as a kid growing up in South Bend who played a lot of golf, I remember him as not one of the warmest people I knew. He was generally stern and had a reputation of telling people when he wasn't happy about something. He was all business.

He walked up to the receptionist's window and gave his name to her. He said that his wife received a call at home from the office saying that, "It was time for his physical." But there was something that he found strange and was puzzled about—he wasn't a patient of my father. He didn't look particularly happy.

The receptionist became wide-eyed. He, indeed, was not my father's patient who she tried to contact for the appointment. Same name, wrong person. There apparently were two people in town with the same name, and she had called the wrong one. She very apologetically explained what had happened. "Is he going to chew her out?" she thought.

"Well," he grumbled, "since I'm here, I might as well get the physical."

11

Did You Notice She Was Wearing a Sweater?

A number of the family practice stories contained in this book attest to the fact that years ago, doctors relied on their physical diagnosis skills much more than they do today. Careful, close observation of the patient and knowing what to look for was extremely important and valuable in the care of their patients. Physicians could not rely on technology such as MRIs and CT scans, and the other expanded radiological and laboratory tests available now.

The author recalls the following episode while a senior medical student rotating with his father, Max Feldman, in South Bend:

While I was making morning rounds with my father, we visited an older woman in her hospital room. She was wearing a sweater. She was admitted for some reason or another and was doing fine. She was close to being discharged and was sitting comfortably in a chair reading a book. She looked up from her book, smiled and greeted us.

"Good morning, Doctor Feldman," she said in a somewhat croaky voice.

My father said hello and introduced me. Like most of the doctors and patients we encountered during rounds, she said something to the effect that she hoped that I would become as good a doctor as my father. I always responded that I could only hope to be.

My father examined her and discussed his continued treatment plans with her. We left the room, and as we were walking down the hall, my father suddenly stopped in his tracks!

He asked me, "Did you notice that woman was wearing a sweater? It's the middle of the summer!" I actually hadn't. It must have been July or August and it was hot and sticky as it usually is in the summertime in Indiana.

"And did you notice her voice?" he reflected. "It's croaky, don't you think?" I actually hadn't noticed that either.

We turned around and proceeded back into her room. "One more thing, if you don't mind me asking. Why are you wearing a sweater?"

She responded, "I always seem to be cold."

He carefully examined her ankle reflexes. They were very slow to recoil—a classic sign of hypothyroidism. He ordered blood tests and, indeed, she was hypothyroid as my father suspected. But he really didn't need the test to know that.

12

When a Doctor Does Not Want to Be Found

My father, Max Feldman, was a hardworking, dedicated family physician who loved his work; he loved medicine and loved seeing his patients. He would work long hours, at times come home late for dinner, and often leave again in the evening to see patients urgently.

But like any self-respecting physician, he loved to play golf. He would take Wednesday afternoons off to pursue this important pastime, as well as Saturday afternoons and Sunday mornings. The time dedicated to golf was almost sacred.

Growing up, I had the opportunity to fill vacancies in my father's regular foursomes. One day, while walking down the fairway with my dad, I told him about some new technology. It was called "the pager." I described it to him explaining that this little device would beep when someone needed him. Some models even had voice capabilities so he could be told exactly what he was needed for. It was a convenient way for the doctor's answering service or the hospital to get a hold of him.

In response to learning about this exciting new technological advancement, my father said, "Now why would I want anyone to find me on the golf course?" He gave me an astonished look, turned away, addressed his ball, and chipped the ball onto the green.

When cell phones were developed, I didn't bother to repeat the conversation.

13

December 7, 1941

Many of the doctors interviewed for this book were World War II veterans. They served in various parts of the world in assorted capacities and settings. Some served as military physicians fresh out of medical school. We can be proud that Hoosier physicians served their country with distinction during this great conflict. Here is one such story of a Hoosier family doctor during the war:

In 1937 my father, Max Feldman, returned to America from medical school in Basil, Switzerland. He then served two years in rotating internships in New York City. Serving an internship was just that—an educational experience and little more. His first year at Lincoln Hospital he earned fifteen dollars per month, and during his second year at the U.S. Public Health Service Hospital on Staten Island, he earned $1,200 a year. Of course, he was provided with small living quarters, a white uniform, and all the food he could eat.

It was 1939 and the Great Depression was at its tail end prior to the United States entry into World War II. It was a time when it took a lot of money to open a private general practice, and it usually took at least five years to successfully establish a practice.

His next steps were financial ones. To have the opportunity to make more money, dad joined the U.S. Army Reserves and also the Civilian Conservation Corps as a camp physician. He was ready for a

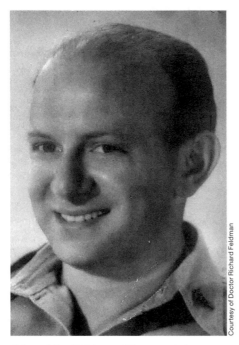

Courtesy of Doctor Richard Feldman

Major Max Feldman, Hawaii, 1941

little adventure and he loved the outdoors. He was offered an assignment in Deaver, Wyoming, near Yellowstone National Park. It was an isolated, dry, and bleak place. It was frigid in the winter with temperatures dipping to minus thirty degrees. There was no social life. The men in the camp were working on large irrigation projects for farming sugar beets and alfalfa. He was the only doctor in the camp, caring for about two hundred men, and he was also in charge of the camp's sanitation. He described it as much like the experience of a military medical officer taking care of a company in an isolated situation. After a long year in northern Wyoming, he was ready for a change.

Being in the reserve, he was obligated to the army for one year of active duty and decided it was a good time to activate. In July 1940 he was assigned to Fort Francis E. Warren in Cheyenne, Wyoming, as the regimental physician. He was the only medical officer at the fort, supervising about forty medics. In September he met an attractive Cheyenne woman, and they were married in November. The marriage lasted sixty-two years.

War was brewing and the military was expanding, and the number of medics at the fort enlarged to about a hundred. A physician captain was brought in as commanding officer and my father said lightheartedly, "I went from chief to nothing!"

As the possibility of war escalated, all reserves serving their year on active duty were "frozen," and he was assigned to Fort Leonard Wood in Missouri and then to Fort Leavenworth in Kansas. He decided to apply for transfer to Hawaii. It was the dream job, and he got it. My father and mother arrived in Honolulu in July 1941. My father was assigned as a ward officer at Tripler Army Hospital.

"Life in Hawaii was a paradise," my mother said, "absolutely a paradise. We were living right on the ocean beach at first, and then we moved to a house with a park nearby that was just beautiful. On the ocean the dolphins performed. Of course, there were also army affairs; we went to dinners where they had singing performances and Hawaiian programs. It was very pleasant." But things changed suddenly.

At five minutes to 8:00 on Sunday morning, December 7, my father was making early rounds at the hospital when he heard explosions. The newspaper commented on the fact there were to be maneuvers that morning. He thought they were louder and more intense than the usual maneuvers, but he did not imagine that Pearl Harbor was being attacked by the Japanese.

My mother was at home at that moment, and trays and dishes were rattling on the shelves. Rushing outside she saw Japanese planes, lots of them, flying low overhead. Friends remarked to her that the planes had the Rising Sun painted on their sides and wings. Dogfights ensued right over her head.

My father also saw planes above. Some were Japanese, but also the remnants of the American squadrons not destroyed at the bombardment at Hickam Field. A few heroic American fighter pilots managed to get off the ground to meet the invaders.

At Tripler Hospital, the staff did not comprehend what actually was transpiring until the casualties started to come through the hospital doors. As my father recounted, "It was the real thing. We were completely surprised; Oahu was being attacked. We were completely unprepared. We didn't expect this. The Japanese could have taken Hawaii without any problem."

The dead, the dying, and the severely injured were pouring into the hospital, both civilian and military. My father had never seen anything like this before in his medical career. Nothing close. Triage medicine had to be employed with so many severely wounded people. He learned about this heartbreaking protocol for mass-casualty military situations, but now he was living it. It was horrific. He was treating people with all kinds of wounds, some catastrophic. All physician officers were on lockdown in the hospital. My father was constantly on duty day and night for two weeks. They were also anticipating another attack and more casualties.

My mother and the other military wives were quickly relocated to high ground above Honolulu. She remembers from that high vantage point observing the remainder of the bombing of Pearl Harbor. It was a poignant and surreal sight.

My Dad recalled, "The bombing only lasted two hours. The army installations were occasionally fired on, but not really bombed. Tripler Hospital was strafed with holes visible on its outside walls. Our car, parked outside of our house, got some shrapnel wounds probably from the dogfights overhead."

There was great anxiety that the island would be invaded. My mother recounted, "Immediately after we were attacked, we went into blackouts, complete blackouts. You wouldn't even dare to light a cigarette outside, because there were no lights whatsoever. We had to cover the bottom of the doorways and tar paper the windows to make sure no light would go through. At night, it was complete blackout, which was quite a contrast to the life we had experienced."

Knowing that their parents would be worried about their safety, my mother called Western Union to send telegrams to Max's parents in New York and her parents in Cheyenne. Communications were ordered to be shut down, and she begged the man there to send them. Western Union finally agreed and sent the telegrams. Shortly thereafter, she called to confirm that they were actually sent after hearing on the radio that all communications had already closed down. She was told, "We are not giving out any information." A few minutes later she called again and kept nagging him for a confirmation. Finally, he verified that they were sent. My mother always believed that her telegrams were the last to be sent from Hawaii after the attack.

My mother and the other military wives were evacuated on February 21, 1942. My father saw her off from the dock. When the ship pulled away, my father took his pack of cigarettes and threw them into the sea. He never smoked again. They were escorted in a convoy of several ships that zigzagged their way to San Francisco. The conditions were terrible. The ship was overcrowded with nine women to a room that was ordinarily meant for two. There were no mattresses except for people who were ill. Since my mother was pregnant, she was one of the lucky ones given a mattress to sleep on. She complained that food was rationed, and it was difficult to get enough to eat, especially for a pregnant woman. My mother believed that during the journey, a torpedo was fired at the convoy but missed.

My mother delivered her first child two weeks after she arrived back in the United States. My father did not see his new son (my older brother) until he was ten months old. When Max finally got leave and came home, mom said to her son, "This is Daddy." Well, this wasn't daddy. Daddy was a picture on the wall.

Major Max Feldman remained in the army until March 1946. From Hawaii he was sent to Christmas Island, a mid-Pacific stopover for military planes from Hawaii to other South Pacific islands. From there he returned to Fort Warren in Cheyenne and then to Fort Leavenworth in Kansas. At Fort Leavenworth, among other duties, he served as the medical officer for a German prisoner-of-war camp. He received that assignment because he was fluent in German.

I remember my father telling me that one day a German prisoner said to him, "Europe is an impenetrable fortress that will never fall." I'm sure my father politely cast some doubt on that pronouncement.

On September 9, 1942, my father wrote in his diary:

The idea of keeping a diary entered my mind some time prior to my departure from Hawaii to Christmas Island. . . . I am indeed sorry that I had not kept the diary from the onset of the War [in] December. For since then, numerous and important occurrences and impressions were experienced which would have had a far greater value had they been put down on paper [then, rather] than a description of them in retrospect . . . such impressions as the sound produced by the bombing of Oahu, the first blackout, the discovery of how great a difference it makes to night visibility whether the moon is out or not, the row upon row of corpses following the Hickam Field bombardment; the bravery with which the causalities that lived suffered their shocking injuries. These and many more occurrences were of such [a] nature as to make a deep impression on [my] mind. In addition to my duties as medical inspector of this post, I have this date also been appointed . . . censor. I censor the enlisted men's mail. I find it interesting, for it gives me an idea of what goes on in the American soldiers' mind. It is an experience that I am thankful for. . . . I never realized how deeply religion can [affect] the personality, character and morality of a person until I took up this job as censor. Now I would be a lot more careful in dealing with our enlisted men, [lest] I hurt anyone's religious feelings. This job has made me change towards my enlisted men. I realize more and more the diversity of character and therefore am inclined to treat each soldier more as an individual than as a group.

On October 7, 1942, he wrote:

The war seems to have taken on favorable turn for the Allies. The Russians are holding (the main front) and on the secondary fronts the Allies are doing well. I am turning optimistic. My opinion is that in 1943, the [Allies] will launch a many front offensive and by the summer of 1944, this horrible war will be over.

My father's prediction wasn't quite correct, but that impenetrable European fortress proved to be vulnerable.

I recall that a number of years ago, a popular Hollywood motion picture was produced on the bombing of Pearl Harbor. Despite the rave reviews, dad scoffed and said, "I don't like seeing movies about Pearl Harbor. They just aren't realistic. The movie was terrible. They didn't capture how horrible that day really was. They couldn't."

My father did not talk much about the war unless he was asked. However, without question, it indelibly affected his life and values; his medical practice; and the way he viewed marriage, family, and the world.

He was, indeed, of that Greatest Generation.

This account was based on the author's reminiscences of discussions with his father, his father's wartime diary, and formal recorded and written interviews conducted by others in 1982 and 2001.

14

A Lesson in Professionalism

Concern has risen within the medical profession about maintaining its long tradition of professionalism in this era of escalating pressures and regulations, decreasing reimbursement, and the increasing corporate and business-like ethic dominating the health-care industry. There is continual apprehension regarding medicine becoming increasingly depersonalized and fragmented. And with that, pride within the profession may easily erode in the process. Doctor Max Feldman was fortunate to have practiced at a time when medicine was simpler and more personal.

When the author was in medical school, he had the treasured opportunity to spend a month rotation with his father. Here is a lesson in professionalism that he learned from him:

One day we saw a patient in his office who couldn't afford to pay for my father's services. He already owed a sizable amount, but my father continued to see him and his family for their medical needs. Walking out of the exam room after seeing this patient, dad's receptionist waved me over to talk with her. She quietly told me, "Your father arranged for this patient to pay five dollars a month on his account." Shaking her head from side to side, she continued, "It costs the office more than five dollars to collect this small payment every month."

That evening, I asked my father why he created an arrangement that made no business sense. He looked a little surprised and then replied, "Richard, it isn't about the money. What's more important is to maintain this patient's sense of self-worth and dignity." That day I learned a valuable lesson from my father.

Coming home from school when I was growing up, I occasionally would find a man working on a special project in our yard or on a home maintenance project. For some patients, it was the only way for them to pay for my father's services. Sometimes, I wondered if the work being done at our home was all that necessary. My father loved and took great pride in his profession, and he cared about the people he served. It's called professionalism.

15

The Tooth

One last story that the author's father told him many years ago:

One day a young boy and his mother urgently made an appointment to see my father in his office. The child had severe abdominal pain that had moved from the middle of his stomach to the right lower area of his abdomen. Along with a history of fever and vomiting, it was a classic presentation of appendicitis. My father told the boy's mother that he was going to admit him to the hospital to have a surgeon perform an appendectomy as soon as possible. He assured her that he would assist in the surgery.

The mother inquired, "What causes an appendicitis, Doctor Feldman?" My father explained that the appendix is a very short, narrow extension of the bowel. Occasionally, something gets caught inside the appendix, causing an obstruction that leads to inflammation and infection. It might have been something such as a seed, a popcorn hull, or something similar. The child's mother immediately responded, "Oh, I think I know exactly what happened! Last week he swallowed a baby tooth. I'll bet that's what got caught in his appendix."

My father thought to himself, "What are the odds of that?" He answered her, "Well, it's possible but unlikely."

The operation went very well. But sure enough, when they removed the appendix and examined it in the surgical pan, out popped the tooth.

16

A Very Important Piece of Equipment

William Wells, MD, was born on December 20, 1930, and was raised in La Porte County, Indiana. After graduating from Indiana University in 1952 with a bachelor of science degree, he attended the IU School of Medicine, graduating in 1956. He traveled to Lima Memorial Hospital in Ohio for his internship, which he completed in 1957. After this internship, he served with the U.S. Air Force as a flight surgeon until 1959, when he entered private practice.

Wells worked as a solo physician for forty years and has been employed by a hospital for twelve years. His practice has included obstetrics and inpatient hospital work. Wells continues to practice in Princeton, Indiana.

As a family doctor during the golden era of family medicine, Wells knew that his patients were more than just patients. They were friends, neighbors, and family members. Going above and beyond to help a patient came naturally to him, and he did it without a second thought. Perhaps it is this attitude that led one particular patient of his to go out of her way to help him one day. Or, perhaps she was just the tiniest bit confused:

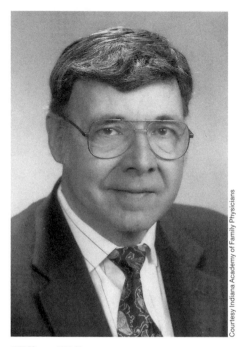

William Wells

Courtesy Indiana Academy of Family Physicians

One thing that happened every so often when I was looking in a patient's ear was that, when I took the scope away—uh-oh! The little plastic speculum stayed in the ear. That little piece comes off so easily, that it's really not that uncommon for that to happen. Well, doctors know that that piece is just something to cover up the scope so you aren't sticking the same piece of equipment in everybody's ear. But there was one little old lady I saw who had a different idea.

She was just a sweet little old lady I saw regularly. One time when she was in for a visit, I looked in one of her ears, and then the other, and that little plastic piece got left behind in her second ear. Whoops! I didn't notice it and, at the time, neither did she. She left the office and went home.

About an hour later, though, she came back in. She had her hands clenched together very determinedly, and she walked up to the front desk.

"Oh, here you go dear," she said very gently to the nurse as she opened her hand carefully, making sure not to drop what she was holding. "I found this in my ear and I know that the doctor's really going to need it. So I brought it back."

The nurse looked at the little piece of plastic for a moment, and then took it very carefully into her own hand. I happened to come out of a room at that point and the nurse told me what the old lady said.

"Oh my goodness. Thank you so much," I told her, "for bringing back that very important piece of equipment!"

We didn't ever have the heart to tell her that as soon as she left that piece went right in the wastebasket!

17

House Call Companion

Back when family doctors made house calls, they did not get to pick and choose when they made those house calls. Sometimes it was raining, sometimes it was snowing, and sometimes it was very, very cold. It just depended on when patients needed their doctors. And if the doctor's car was not quite equipped to handle the elements, well, the doctor had to go anyway. He just had to find ways of adjusting. Doctor Wells found very creative ways of handling those late-night house calls:

I had a Volkswagen in those days. It was a beautiful blue 1959 Volkswagen, just about three years old. A pretty looking car. I always took it when I was out making house calls. Well, I didn't know this when I bought it, but it turns out the old Volkswagens might not have really been built for a doctor making house calls in the middle of the night. They didn't have heaters.

They had manifold heaters, but you would have had to drive all the way to Evansville to get that going. I live in Princeton, so I was always making house calls when it was freezing cold—in and out of my car.

Now, going out to make a house call at three in the morning, which

I did in a cold Volkswagen with no heater, would normally be pretty unbearable. But I had something that a lot of physicians didn't have. I had Ebineezer.

Ebineezer was just a monstrous yellow cat that lived in a little nook above the garage in our house, where it was warm. Every time without fail, when he heard me turn on the car in the middle of the night, he would come down his little walkway into the garage, crawl in that Volkswagen, and get on my lap and make house calls with me. There's really nothing like a warm cat on your lap in the middle of the winter at three o'clock in the morning.

Well, besides maybe a working heater—but I wasn't that lucky!

18

Of Horses and Buggies

William Blaisdell, MD, was born August 26, 1934, and was raised in Roll, Indiana. He attended Purdue University, receiving a bachelor of science in 1956. Subsequently, he taught vocational agriculture and chemistry at Tyner and Walkerton High Schools in Indiana.

Blaisdell received a Reserve Officers' Training Corps commission from the U.S. Army Reserve program at Purdue and served on active duty and also commanded a reserve unit at Argos, Indiana. In 1965 he graduated from the Indiana University School of Medicine and served a rotating internship at Brooke Army Medical Center in San Antonio, Texas.

Blaisdell began a family medicine practice in Seymour, Indiana, in July 1966 as a solo physician. Since then, he has established a group practice that now has a total of six family physicians, two nurse practitioners, and a physician's assistant. His present scope of practice includes general medicine and endoscopy. During the initial forty-four years of practice, Blaisdell also provided obstetrical care and was a member of the anesthesia department at Schneck Medical Center in Seymour, Indiana. He is a Fellow of the American Academy of Family Physicians. Here Blaisdell recalls a time gone by in family medicine:

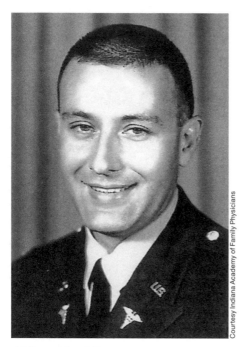

Courtesy Indiana Academy of Family Physicians

William Blaisdell

There was a doctor in town named Bud Grassley. He had started a general practice in 1918.

Doctor Grassley's father was a physician before him in this town. He started sometime in the 1800s. So, Bud liked to fish, and he had a pond on a farm out north of town. Well, I like to fish, so we got together and occasionally we'd fish together.

One day, we're fishing out on his pond, and he said to me that his dad told him there was something that he could never practice medicine without. And he wanted to see if I knew what that could be.

I thought a minute, and said, "No, I don't think I know what that could be."

He said, "A good horse."

Well back then, his dad practiced out of a buggy. So he needed a horse, but Doctor Grassley said that he never needed one as did his father.

Editor's Note: The transition to the automobile had taken place by 1918. A country doc with his horse and buggy is part of our archetypal image of those bygone days.

19

The Illusive Hernia

I'll tell you another Doctor Grassley story. When I was first in practice, I was seeing a patient in the emergency room. The patient was a little infant who was inconsolable, crying, and thrashing. Obviously, he was sick.

I looked this child over carefully, but I couldn't find a real obvious reason for the infant's condition. I really couldn't find anything. So about that time, I saw Doctor Grassley coming down the hallway, with a cigar in his mouth. Not lit, just in his mouth. Doctor Grassley performed surgery in his general practice. Actually, he did the first bowel resection in this town.

I said, "Hey, would you mind taking a look at this child? I'm puzzled about it." Of course he said he would.

He took a look at this child and stepped back into the hallway and said, "I think the child has an incarcerated right groin hernia."

I said, "What makes you think he has an incarcerated hernia? I didn't see a hernia!"

"You can't see the hernia but the right testicle is retracted." He had observed a very subtle diagnostic sign. The testicle was being pulled up by the hernia or by a muscular reflex secondary to the pain.

I anesthetized the kid, and during surgery we, indeed to everyone's surprise, found an incarcerated hernia. This is a good example of how the old docs figured things out. They didn't have CT scanners, or fancy technology. But they became exceedingly observant. They were masters of physical diagnosis. They were great diagnosticians.

Editor's Note: Reading this account today is somewhat puzzling. A retracted testicle is not generally part of the clinical picture of an incarcerated hernia. But every clinical situation is different and some unique. The old doctor's diagnostic skills and intuition from years of experience proved to be precise in this unusual situation.

20

Beyond the Usual Call of Duty

Occasionally family doctors are needed for assistance beyond the call of their usual medical duties. In special circumstances, what is expected is not medical expertise but just being a friend, as Blaisdell would find out one evening with a patient in Seymour, Indiana.

He [the patient] used to like to fish out on the White River all the time. It was August, the time of the year when the catfish bite.

Blaisdell and his patient set up baits all along the river the evening before in hopes of a victorious catch the next day. But with the odds probably against them.

The next morning, I met him out there, and we went to bait after bait, and nothing. Then, we came to the last one we had set, and this line was tearing and shaking. We were sure there was something big on it. We pulled this line up, and here comes the largest fish I'd ever seen. It turned out to be a forty-five-pound catfish. Well, my friend said, "He's about to tear off." So, he put his hand in the catfish's mouth, grabbed it, and asked me to cut the line. I took out my pocket knife and cut the line. Now we were going down the river in this ten-foot boat nearly up on its side trying to pull the fish in. Well, he couldn't pull it in. He didn't have enough strength to fight the fish. My friend had bib overalls on and his hard hat. He was in the middle of this boat kneeling over the side holding onto this fish. I got behind him and on the count of three, I pulled on his bib overalls, he pulled on the fish, and then the fish came into the boat. Now we had two men and one mad catfish in a ten-foot boat.

Of course, Blaisdell and his patient were compelled to share their victory with the community.

It was end of summer, so we took the catfish down to the county fair and put it in a live tank they had there. A guy came along and asked to buy the catfish. My friend sold the catfish for fifteen bucks, and the guy took the catfish home and put it in his pond. As far as I know, the catfish could still be there.

21

A Desperate Move

Knowing that a young patient before him was going to die, Blaisdell tried a desperate measure to save this girl's life.

Sometime in the 1960s, there was this sixteen-year-old patient of mine who developed abdominal pain, and it turned out to be a ruptured appendix. She is still in my practice today. She became septic, which means she was infected and had bacteria in her bloodstream. It appeared that she was going to die.

She was in shock, and we could hardly sustain her blood pressure. Of course in those days, we didn't have an ICU. We were doing what we could do, running fluids and the usual antibiotics we had at the time.

So, I heard there was a new class of antibiotics known as aminoglycosides. I heard that this drug was coming, but it had not been approved and released by the FDA [Food and Drug Administration]. Well, I called the company in New York State, and I explained the situation. I told them that she was infected with an organism for which I had no effective antibacterial agent. I understood they were going to market this drug and asked if it was far enough along that they would consider giving it to us.

They said yes, and they had the drug flown to the Indianapolis airport. The State Police picked up the drug and raced it down the road.

I remember sitting by her bedside that night at nine o'clock thinking she would never survive the night. She was unconscious. Her blood pressure was barely detectable. I pushed that drug in IV, and the next morning she was talking to me.

Aminoglycosides are still in use today and still save a lot of lives. I must have been one of the first to use it in practice!

Editor's Note: Antibiotics were, indeed, one of the medical miracles of the twentieth century. One wonders that with all of today's regulations and governmental bureaucracy if procuring an unapproved drug in a critical situation would even be possible.

22

It's Just the Way It Was

Before anesthesiologists were routinely available, especially in small towns, family doctors often performed surgical anesthesia for their patients. Unfortunately years ago, anesthesia was given without the safety and monitoring advancements and technology we enjoy today. Blaisdell recounts:

You couldn't find anyone who wanted be an anesthesiologist in a small community. So of course, doctors like me did all the anesthesia. And so for my first thirty-seven years of my practice, I was on call every third to fifth night depending on how many people needed it.

I like anesthesia. I like the science of it; I like the skills it requires.

Back when I trained, because we didn't have anesthesiologists in small communities, it was expected that family docs would learn enough about anesthesia to do it safely. But the agents we had to use were pretty archaic by modern standards. We didn't have electronic monitoring and we didn't have mechanical ventilators. We couldn't measure oxygen saturations, and we didn't have any idea what the carbon dioxide level was.

There was a rather routine surgical case of a roughly thirty-five-year-old woman. The only monitor you had at that time for the heart was to keep your finger on the pulse. So, I would routinely sit there breathing for the patient by squeezing a bag, and at the same time I kept one finger on the pulse. I was also running this anesthetic, which was notorious for causing cardiac irregularities. But this agent was the first step up from ether. All of a sudden, this patient's heart stopped in one beat. So we resuscitated her, and shocked her out of it, changed the anesthetic, and she was just fine.

But the point is, you were subject to those kinds of things all the time. Back then that's just the way it was. Later, when we told the patient what had happened, as I recall, she just sort of casually said, "Well, everything's all right." Everything was.

23

The Attack

A small-town family doctor could often treat a patient in the emergency room with a serious illness. But on this rare occasion, Blaisdell was suddenly presented with "a load" of patients with a common, but not so serious condition.

I was on call one night in the 1960s. I was down in the emergency room seeing a patient of mine the night of a regional basketball tournament, which was being played here in Seymour. All of a sudden, this flood of patients came in. I mean a flood.

What had happened was someone had set off tear gas on the Scottsburg team and student buses. I was sure it was tear gas. It just had to be. But the school administrator was certain the kids had all been poisoned.

So, I had three busloads of kids, the coaches, and the basketball team in the emergency room. They were all hysterical; they also were sure they'd been poisoned. Well, I'd been in the military, so I knew from experience that it was tear gas, and although they didn't feel so good, it really wasn't all that serious.

What a scene! I had to convince all these people that no one was going to die. But you know, they weren't so sure. I had all these kids hyperventilating and wailing and pacing. It took all night to get everyone calmed down.

I don't even remember who won the game.

24

Naked Ladies

Paul Macri, MD, was born December 4, 1934. He was raised in Mishawaka, Indiana, where he graduated from Mishawaka High School in 1953. He earned his undergraduate degree from Wabash College, graduating in 1957. Macri attended the Indiana University School of Medicine, graduating in 1961. He completed a rotating internship at Marion County General Hospital before entering practice in 1962.

Macri worked as a solo physician and served as the team physician for Mishawaka High School from 1968 to 1995. He had a wide scope of practice, including obstetrics, minor surgery, and orthopedics. Macri also served on the faculty at the IU School of Medicine regional campus at the University of Notre Dame as a volunteer clinical assistant professor. Although he retired from medicine in 1998, he continues to treat some patients.

Seeing people without their clothes on is, of course, a part of a physician's profession. Being a daily occurrence, doctors come to consider it routine and just do not think about it much, except in certain contexts as Macri's story points out:

I remember one night when I was an intern. It was late July and one of those hot, steamy, sticky Indiana nights. One of those nights where

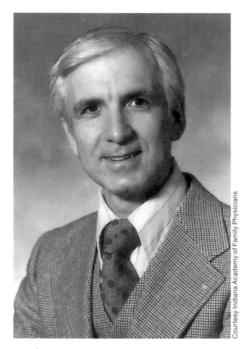

Courtesy Indiana Academy of Family Physicians

Paul Macri

you can just feel the humidity cover you all the time, no matter where you go, like a thick blanket you can't take off. Just hot, hot, hot.

I was working OB service that night, which basically meant that when a pregnant lady would come up, I would examine her. I would do a pelvic exam, and I would listen to the baby's heart. There were about six women staying at the hospital that night, all pregnant, just waiting for their time to come; they were all due to deliver in the next day or two. We had them all staying in the same room, six beds—two rows of three, like a room at summer camp or in a sorority.

Because it was so unbearably hot, I'm sure you can imagine they were a little uncomfortable, a little ornery. And when it comes to a pregnant woman—let alone a room full of six of them—you let them do what they need to do. That's something I learned very quickly in my internship: There is no bossing around a pregnant woman in labor.

So, in order to feel more comfortable in the heat, the women had taken all their clothes off, and were naked in their beds except for a sheet covering them. And they were there all night complaining of labor pains and their discomfort, and they'd kick off the sheets. So there you go. A room full of six naked women, lying in their beds.

So it's late at night, it must have been midnight or one in the morning. I walk up to see how my patient is doing. On the stairwell, I see three of my intern cohorts all crowded around a window with their faces pressed against the glass looking outside. They looked like little kids with their noses pressed against the window of a chocolate shop.

"What are you guys looking at?" I asked.

"Shh!" they barked back.

"Come over here," one of them whispered, without taking his eyes off the window.

I came over.

"Just quiet down and look over there," he told me.

I looked, but I didn't see anything.

"That's the nurses' dorm over there," another one explained. "I think we can see them taking a shower."

"You've got to be kidding me," I said.

Here they had a room full of women who were stark-raving nude, and they're crowded around a tiny 1 x 2 foot window trying to catch a glimpse of the student nurses over there.

I guess it's just a matter of perspective. There was no connection in their minds between their imagination about the nurses over there and these six women in the room next door to them. They were patients, so they just didn't think about it.

25

Miracle Baby

After years of clinical experience, prudent doctors come to understand that quick decisions do not always render the best results. Patience, careful consideration, and giving the case a little time to unfold can be the best medicine, as Macri explains:

I remember one story very vividly from when I was working OB. I heard the nurses in the ER talking about a woman who was not a patient of mine. She was from Elkhart, and she was about two months pregnant. She had called the ER because she started bleeding, pretty heavily. It sounded like she was miscarrying. She was scared, and she wanted to know what to do. The nurses told her they recommended a D and C, which is a procedure where you scrape the lining of the uterus. It makes the hemorrhaging stop by removing a pregnancy that has gone badly.

I said, "I couldn't help overhearing your conversation, and it seems like this patient is really scared and worried. Could I talk to her on the phone?"

They said sure you can. So I called the woman, and I explained to her the procedure they wanted to do to stop the bleeding, if indeed, it appeared that she was losing the baby. It was around 2 a.m.

"Boy," she said, "do we have to do that? Maybe the bleeding will stop and my baby will be okay."

So, I asked her, "Well is the bleeding quieting down?"

"Yes it is," she said, "I'm not bleeding as much as when I was at the hospital."

So I listened to her, and then I told her we'd do nothing tonight, and that I would see her tomorrow. I trusted that she was telling the truth, and she trusted that I would do everything I could to keep her and her baby safe.

I told the ER nurses about my conversation with the patient, and they kind of wrote off the situation. Since I wasn't planning on doing their procedure, they said, "Well, do what you want, but she's your responsibility now." I said okay.

The next day the patient came in and I saw her, and she was right—the bleeding had lessened considerably. I kept monitoring her and eventually the bleeding stopped entirely. The baby was fine.

Seven months go by, and the woman goes on to have the baby. I delivered it, a beautiful baby girl. We called her the "miracle baby."

After that, the mom and her daughter became regular patients of mine. Every time I saw that baby in the office, I used to think, "Wow, if it were not for that mother's courage and belief that, just maybe, the bleeding would stop, that little miracle baby wouldn't be here.

That's the kind of stuff that's rewarding.

26

A Daughter's Broken Arm

Why is it that physicians commonly minimize the illnesses of their own family members? And when making the decision to treat them, sometimes docs just do not provide the same careful attention they afford their other patients. Macri was guilty of those very things in the following episode:

As a family doctor, I made sacrifices for my career and my patients. But in some ways, it was my family who made the bigger sacrifices. We never went on a vacation for more than a week at a time because I would have women in labor. That was just the way it was. Family paid a price for that. If it wasn't for my wife, I couldn't have done any of the things I did in my career or anything else. I'll be the first to say that it was my wife who raised all five kids. She cooked all the meals; she took the kids to school and did volunteer work in the school. She paid all the bills and took care of all the plumbing and maintenance in our home. And as if that wasn't enough, she helped me at the office too. She oversaw the bookwork; she set up all the records at my office.

Back in those days, if you were a doctor's wife that's just the way it was. Pam was the one who figured out how to be home at 3:00 p.m.

every day when the kids got off school. Every doctor's wife we talked to lived the same life. It was a domestic agreement that was true in most physician homes back then. That isn't true now. In some ways it was good, and in some ways it was bad, but I know one thing for sure: If I hadn't had a good support system—my family and my wife—there's no way I could have done the job that I did. No way.

And like I said, I'm not proud of it, but sometimes my family paid a price for my career. This is one of those stories:

My daughter Lisa, who is a professional dancer now, was in ballet for years. One day she was in school practicing ballet and she fell down and hurt herself. Not terribly, it didn't seem, but we were at home that night and Pam said, "You better take a look at Lisa's arm."

It felt pretty tender, so I took Lisa to get an x-ray of her arm. A friend of mine took the x-ray, so we didn't have to go to the ER.

"Call me and tell me what it looks like," I told my friend.

When he called with the results of the x-ray, he said it looked good, nothing showed up on the x-ray whatsoever.

"It's just a bruise, don't worry about it," I told Lisa.

So the next day Lisa goes to school, and she comes home and complains that her arm still hurts. Next day, the same thing.

Finally my wife, Pam, said, "Paul, if you don't look at her elbow again I'm going to get a second opinion!"

I thought, "Well that's something. A second opinion!"

"But I looked again, and I called my friend who did the x-ray and asked him to look at it again. He said it still looked fine, but told me to send Lisa over to see him again in person. So, I sent Lisa over to see him, and he saw her. When I came in his office, he had some news for me."

"Paul, she's tender far above where the x-ray was," he said. "You ordered an X-ray for her elbow, but her bruise is over her humorous on her upper arm."

He X-rayed her humorous. And guess what? She had a broken arm. She'd had one for five days!

When she came to school the next day wearing her cast, her friends said, "Lisa, didn't you hurt that a week ago? Isn't your dad a doctor?"

"Well, yes he is!" she said. "That's what happens when your dad's a doctor!"

27

The Last Little Girl

Wilbur McFadden, MD, was born on June 7, 1931, and was raised in Ohio. He attended Manchester College in North Manchester, Indiana, graduating with a bachelor of arts degree in 1953. He then studied at the University of Illinois College of Medicine, where he received his medical degree in 1957. After completing an internship and a two-year surgical residency in Michigan, McFadden joined the Manchester Clinic in 1969 and retired in 1999.

Throughout his family medicine career, McFadden worked in a partnership practice that included obstetrics, general surgery, emergency department care, and addiction medicine. He spent seven years in missionary medicine in Puerto Rico and Indonesia.

When Doctor Wilbur McFadden chose to become a family physician, he did so for a number of reasons. Mainly it was because as a family physician, he was able to do a variety of different things and experience the life of his patients in all of its stages, from birth to death. He said, "Choosing a specialty would mean giving something up. I liked it all. Family practice was an opportunity to do it all. I was an

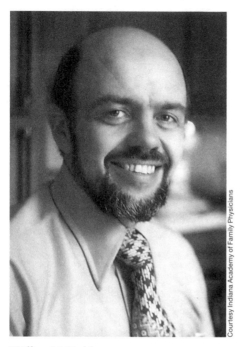

Courtesy Indiana Academy of Family Physicians

Wilbur McFadden

old-fashioned family doctor."

McFadden always had a soft spot in his heart for families. "For the most part, my practice consisted of good people doing good things. Like good parents doing the right things with their children."

One family sticks out in McFadden's memory. He was involved in all of their medical care. "This was a very nice, extraordinarily nice, family. She was a good mother," he recalled.

McFadden delivered three of the children. The family's fourth child, Amy, was born at a hospital in Fort Wayne. She was premature and weighed one pound and nine ounces.

He felt so close to the family that when his nurse died suddenly, he called the mother of this family to explain what happened. "She was very close to my nurse who had helped deliver the babies. She was one of two patients that I called right after Jan, the nurse, had died to let them know what was going on," he said. That was a hard time for him, but he wanted this family to hear about it from him, not just from reading the local newspaper.

Because McFadden had this very special relationship with the family for such a long time, he also considered them when he began thinking about retirement. He told Amy, the youngest, "I will stay in practice long enough to see you go off to kindergarten."

So, he did. His last appointment on the day that he retired was giving Amy her physical to enter into kindergarten. A photograph of that encounter was posted in the local newspaper reporting on his retirement.

It was a very proud but bittersweet moment. McFadden was, as he would say, "an old-fashioned family doctor" who developed close, lasting relationships with his patients and their families. They relied on him, loved him, and invited him into their lives.

28

Third Time's the Charm

Gene Creek, MD, was raised in Evansville, Indiana. He attended Indiana University in Bloomington, receiving a bachelor of arts degree in 1949. Creek continued his education at the IU School of Medicine, earning his medical degree in 1952. He completed postgraduate training at IU before serving in the U.S. Army from 1953 to 1955.

In 1955 Creek began a wide scope of practice that included obstetrics and anesthesia, as well as emphasis on gastrointestinal diseases and endoscopy. In addition, Creek received many academic appointments, including clinical professor at the IU School of Medicine and course director for internal medicine and director of medical education at Bloomington Hospital. Creek retired from his practice in 2008.

There are times when a family doc needs to just offer a small common-sense suggestion to his patients to get them going on a better course of action, as Creek describes:

One of the biggest differences between the practice of medicine now and the practice of medicine when I started out is the insurance companies. When I started practicing family medicine years ago, insurance companies had nowhere near the influence on doctors and patients as they do today. Doctor-patient confidentiality was much more real. You didn't tell the insurance companies everything. Sometimes doctor-patient confidentiality manifested itself in the silliest of ways:

I remember one family I saw regularly. They had seven boys, ages two to fourteen, so I don't need to tell you that they were always in and out of my office because of some trouble the boys were getting into. Hardly a week went by when I didn't see one or the other of them.

There was one of the smaller boys who, at one point, got onto a kick for sticking beans up his nose. Now, he did this three days in a row.

At that time, Blue Cross allowed you to remove a foreign body from a patient's nose only so many times and have them pay for it. I had already taken the beans out of his nose twice in two days, so I thought, "Boy, if I do that a third time they'll be down here investigating me."

So instead of reporting it, I just took out the bean for free that third time, and I didn't tell the insurance company. It was just easier that way.

Well, I told the parents what I had done and gently suggested that maybe they consider trying to take the beans away from their son. Well, the parents looked at me and then at each other. A light went off! And tell you what. It worked pretty well!

29

A Snowy House Call

Almost every family doctor made house calls in the 1950s and 1960s, and usually they were relatively routine. At-home births were not uncommon. Doctors usually knew what to expect, knew where their patients lived, and had no trouble getting to their patients. Well, almost no trouble.

Creek remembers a time when making a house call was just a little bit more challenging than normal:

I made a house call in the middle of a snowstorm one time. And this was no ordinary snowstorm; it was the biggest snow we'd had in years. It was the biggest snow I can remember from all my years as a doctor. It was around 1965, and roads were closed all over town. If this had been something that could wait until the morning, I would have tried to wait and have the patient come to my office. But as it turns out, it couldn't wait—one of my patients was going into labor. Unfortunately, you can't really tell a baby who's on the way to sit tight and wait until some weather passes. You've just got to make do with what you have.

The pregnant woman lived in Monroe County, down on the other side of the causeway from Lake Monroe. She called me saying she was going into labor, and she wasn't able to move. The snow that night was so bad that I didn't think my car would be able to make it out to her. So, I called the state police and they came by to take me down there. But when we got out of town, it turned out not even their police cars could make it—the snow was piling up too fast, and their cars just weren't strong enough.

So, the state police called a snowplow to go ahead of us. It was working pretty well, all things considered, until we got to the causeway. The snow out there was just too deep. It looked like we weren't going to be able to make it out to the pregnant lady's house. The state police couldn't make it, and the snowplow couldn't make it; it wasn't looking good.

I noticed that there was a space just about a foot or two wide between the causeway railing and the road—the only space in sight where the snow wasn't piled up a few feet into the air. It looked just big enough for someone to walk it. So that's what I did.

The causeway was about a half mile, and I'll tell you, it was pretty cold. But I was prepared for it and determined to get there.

To make a long story short, I arrived at the woman's house and she was in labor, but it turned out she wasn't so close that we were going to have to deliver in her home.

So we had a doc, a snowplow, police cars, and a woman in labor. I'll tell you one thing: she had quite an escort to the hospital!

But you know, it was a good feeling to have all that help and concern of others in a difficult situation. Everyone pulled together.

30

The True Use of Boiling Water

Typical of home-delivery scenes in old movies is the doctor urgently asking someone to boil a pot of water. The average movie viewer, however, probably does not know exactly what the boiling water is for—it seems never to be used. Well, as it turns out, real doctors do not even know what the boiling water is for! That is, until one day they learn, as was the case for Creek.

It was 1952 and it was only the second or third delivery that I took care of. It was in downtown Indianapolis, at the corner of Washington and Meridian Streets. It was a hot, sticky day in the middle of July.

I had gotten a call about this delivery that needed to be taken care of in the home—we called this an "outdoor delivery" because it was out of the hospital. I was driving a general hospital car, and outside the clinic where I worked there was a public-health nurse standing there. She looked like she was just leaving her shift or something. This is when nurses still wore all white uniforms and Oxford shoes that tied.

She came up to me as I was going on a delivery and said, "Are you going on a delivery doctor?"

I said I was. She said she'd never been on an outdoor delivery.

So I said, "Honey, I've only seen one or two myself, so come along! I could use any help I could get!"

Once we arrived, we were at the patient's house for probably an hour or so, and the baby came easily. I handed it to the nurse and tied the umbilical cord. I was getting ready to deliver the placenta; but wait, there's a foot hanging out! All of a sudden we had twins.

All I could remember about delivering a baby feet first was what I learned when we practiced with a mannequin in medical school. Needless to say, I was a little nervous. I remembered that the big secret was "don't do anything—just let nature take its course!" You were supposed to follow that rule unless you think the cord is stuck, which could easily happen since the baby is coming out the opposite direction. You've got a time limit, and if you wait too long the baby might not make it.

Well, the second baby came out but there was one problem: When I handed the second baby over, there was nothing to tie the cord with.

So what we had was a nurse, and we had boiling water. Now, how do you get the cord tied?

Apparently, you take the nurse's shoe strings! I didn't know this up to that time, but the nurse did. She took the string off one of her shoes. We boiled it, and we tied the cord with it.

So, those pots of boiling water you see in the old movies? I still don't know what the water is for. But, that's the use I found for it!

31

A Loaded Diagnosis

When Creek was practicing family medicine it was not uncommon for him to look after other doctors' patients when they left town for vacations or family commitments. Now, even though he did not have a long history with these patients, he was still usually able to earn their trust and help them. He recalls, however, one patient who had a little bit of trouble trusting him after one incident.

I remember one woman who came in to see me when her doctor was out of town. She taught school over in Brown County, a nice seeming lady. She had a kidney infection. I saw her for a regular visit, took her history, took a urine sample for analysis, diagnosed her problem, and treated her.

I had her return a week later after her urine analysis came back, and I spoke with her about how she was feeling. Her urinary symptoms were gone and she was feeling fine. I didn't hear from her again.

When her regular doctor came back to town, she went back to him and said, "That Doctor Creek—well, I won't be returning to him. Not for any reason!"

He asked her what was wrong and she said, "Well doctor, he called me a drunk."

"He said it to your face?" the doctor asked.

"No, but I saw him write it on the chart. And doctor, I've never had a drink in my life!"

The whole thing seemed a little fishy to the doctor, so he called me about it. I couldn't figure out what the patient could have been referring to; I really had no idea. He told me that she said she'd seen me write on the chart that she was "loaded."

Oh boy, I thought. I had written that after all, but I'd meant her urine analysis. It was the thing that was loaded—loaded with pus cells!

32

They Know Where to Find You

Eldon Baker, MD, was born on April 4, 1930, in Quinter, Kansas. He received his bachelor of arts in 1952 from the University of Kansas. He continued at the university for his medical degree, which he earned in 1955. Baker completed an internship at Kansas City General Hospital. Baker has been licensed in four states, including Kansas, Pennsylvania, Maryland, and Indiana, where he began practicing in 1958. His private practice was located in Delphi, and he admitted patients at Saint Elizabeth Hospital and Home Hospital, both in Lafayette. He maintained his private practice until 1996 and then volunteered at the Riggs Community Health Center, serving low-income and uninsured individuals and families, until 2006. Baker is now retired and lives in Delphi.

When Baker began practicing medicine, not only was there no email or cell phone, there were no answering machines. His patients could call his office to schedule an appointment, but if nobody was in, they simply had to call back. (Though, Baker was "in" a lot more often than today's doctors are.) Unless, of course, somebody tracked him down. More often than not, the friendly neighborhood operators were the ones who knew just where to find him.

When I first came to town, the way somebody got in contact with you was to call the operator. The operators worked at huge switchboards with little wires they'd plug in to connect one person to another. It really was just like in the movies you see today.

Well, my wife and I were at our friends' house for dinner one night, and the telephone rang. My friend answered it and got a funny look on his face.

"It's for you," he told me.

I answered, and the operator said she had a call for me from one of my patients.

"Well okay," I said, "but how did you know I would be here?"

"It's Thursday," she replied. "You always eat with the Johnsons on Thursdays!" It was a great system, really. The operators got a sense of my schedule and of the places I frequently went. Sometimes I would let them know if I was going out, but often I forgot to tell them. It was probably because I knew in my head that they would find ways to hunt me down and find me anyway! These girls would just be sharp enough to figure out where we were likely to be and put the calls through to that place.

When we went to a full dial system we tried to get by with a telephone answering device at my office. Now, that worked better than not having an answering device, I suppose. But to this day no technology I've encountered has worked better than those operators who could hunt the doctors down just by their own intuition!

33

The Smell of Smallpox

Baker was often given the opportunity to learn the profession of family practice from his predecessors in town. Some of the information he gleaned from them was, incidentally, not the kind of things he had learned in medical school. Baker remembers one of these lessons clearly; it was a lesson about a doctor's instinct:

When I started here in Delphi it was 1958, and there were a handful of doctors in town who, as was the custom, had spent their whole careers in town. One of them was a doctor who was eighty-something years old, but he was still just as active as he had always been and went to his office every day of the week. This doctor was interesting in that he had been in town for a very long time, and he was the only person in the whole area that had ever seen a smallpox patient. All the other physicians would call on him at different times to see their patient when smallpox was suspected.

He used to talk about the time they wanted him to come down to the hospital at Lafayette to determine if a patient had smallpox or not. So, he got in his car and he drove down to Lafayette from Delphi and arrived at this hospital prepared to diagnose this patient.

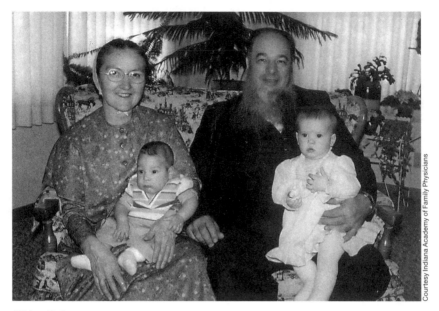

Courtesy Indiana Academy of Family Physicians

Eldon Baker

Well, he arrived at the hospital, walked into the corridor where the patient in question was supposed to be. As he walked down the corridor he turned to the doctors from Lafayette who were next to him and said, "There's no smallpox here."

"Well, how do you know?" they asked. "You haven't even seen the patient yet."

"I know," the doc said, "because it doesn't smell like smallpox."

He examined the patient and determined the actual diagnosis, and sure enough—no smallpox in that hospital. This is one of the most important differences between the way medicine is practiced today and the way it was when I was starting out. Nowadays, a doctor would have to perform a dozen tests. Back then, it was trust in the clinical skill that comes with experience. He didn't need any tests. He smelled the air and he knew there was no smallpox.

He was right. He knew what he was doing. That sense of intuition and the ability to make a diagnosis just by careful attention to the patient is something that's truly missing today.

34

Lines of Love

*While Baker lived and practiced medicine during the time of tele-
phones, some of his predecessors had to work harder to find ways to keep
in contact with their patients. He remembers a story about a Doctor
Crampton, a Delphi doctor who served as his mentor and inspiration:*

Doctor Crampton was an old doc when I first came to town. He
was kind of a local legend, a great storyteller and a great doc. He was
entirely dedicated to his patients and made sure he did everything he
could for them.

There was one patient of his, a pregnant lady who had to have a
caesarean section. He delivered the baby in her home. Now, this was
in the 1930s and a caesarian section was a riskier procedure then than it
is these days. If a doc performed one, it was the kind of thing where he
would want to make sure he could keep in contact with the patient for
a few days or weeks afterward, to make sure everything was going okay.

Well, a couple problems arose. The patient lived out in the county, pretty far from Doctor Crampton's office. Also, she didn't have a
telephone and there weren't even any telephone lines out there in the

county. Doctor Crampton had no way to get a hold of this patient on a daily basis. So what did he do about this problem?

Doctor Crampton walked the distance between his patient's house and his office, strung telephone wire by hand onto fence posts, and had a telephone installed at the patient's house. That way, he could keep in contact with her every day. You might say he went the "extra mile"!

35

Doctor's Helping Hands, and Sometimes Feet

Daniel Cannon, MD, was born on New Year's Day, 1923. He received his doctor of medicine degree from the University of Louisville in December 1946 before completing a rotating internship at Episcopal Hospital in Philadelphia, Pennsylvania. Cannon entered family practice in February 1947, practicing in New Albany, Indiana. He had a solo practice that focused on obstetrics and surgery. He retired in September 2010.

Cannon taught medical students at Indiana University, the University of Louisville, and the University of Kentucky. He was also the Floyd County Coroner for eighteen years.

Doctor Dan Cannon was asked, "What is the difference between medicine in the old days and medicine now?" He simply says, with a mixture of seriousness and lightheartedness, "We used to examine patients." The time when doctors personally examined, tested, and treated each and every one of their patients without the use of emergency rooms, offsite laboratories, or nurse practitioners—those are the days Doctor Cannon remembers. And those are the days that made him fall in love with medicine.

In those bygone days, doctors couldn't always X-ray a patient to find out what was wrong, Cannon explains, because the "X-ray man" as he puts it, would only come into the hospital a couple times a week. Needless to say, he wasn't always available when a patient needed help with a problem. Family physicians were, more often than not, solely responsible for diagnosing and treating a patient. Cannon remembers a professor in medical school telling him and his classmates that, "If we took a good history and did a good, thorough medical examination, and we didn't know what was wrong with the patient, the chances were nine out of ten that we'd never know."

Patients also relied more on their doctors in the mid-twentieth century, says Cannon. "Patients thought differently about their doctors than they do now." And with good reason. The general practitioner was usually the only one around.

In general, as time went on and the practice of medicine evolved, more and more people—physicians and patients alike—began to rely on ancillary procedures in hospitals or laboratories outside the doctors' offices. "The fine art of practicing medicine isn't being done anymore," Cannon explains. He describes the process of doctors hearing from their patients what's wrong, and then sending them to the laboratory or radiology to have tests done. Today, doctors don't examine the patients nearly as much. As he puts it, "Doctors, in other words, don't lay hands on people anymore."

Today's methods for practicing medicine mark a significant change from the early days of Cannon's practice when it was standard for a doctor to lay hands on his patients. Or, in some rare cases, feet.

Cannon remembers a house call where the patient wanted him to go to any lengths he could to treat her at home:

"I got a telephone call from an elderly lady who had fallen at her home and dislocated her shoulder. When I went out on the call I told her we'd have to go to the hospital and get it X-rayed. Today, that would have been standard procedure. Everybody wants an X-ray now; there's really no two ways about it. But when I told her this she said, 'Oh doctor, I don't want to go to the hospital. Can't you do something about it here?'"

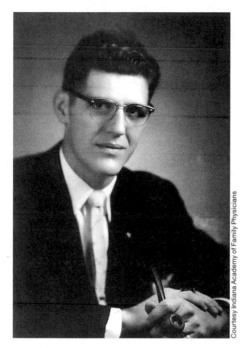

Courtesy Indiana Academy of Family Physicians

Daniel Cannon

"Well, I guess so," I replied.

"Now, back then one of the few drugs we really had for house calls was morphine. You would commonly give it to patients who were in pain. That's part of the reason hospitals are used more these days. If someone called me with a heart attack and asked me to come out, all I had to give them, unfortunately, was morphine, and that's not really the appropriate treatment. Sometimes when you went on a house call, all you could do was check the patient's temperature and make sure they were getting enough rest and fluids. And, maybe you would give them some morphine if they were in pain.

"So, I gave this elderly lady a shot of morphine for her shoulder and waited a few minutes to see if she started feeling any better. She didn't, really. It seemed like she needed something else to relieve the pain. I knew that one of the ways to reduce a dislocated shoulder is to pull on it. If you pull on the arm and shoulder gently, it will stretch the muscles enough that the dislocated shoulder will pop back into place.

"Since she was determined not to take the trip to the hospital, I decided the best thing to do would be to pop her shoulder myself right there. I told her that this was the only way to remedy the problem at home with no equipment like they have in the emergency room. She replied that was just fine. She wanted me to do whatever I could to take care of her at home.

"I fixed her shoulder right there at her home, and you know, she never did get that X-ray. But I'll tell you, she was awful surprised when I took off my shoe and told her, 'Get ready! I'm going to stick my foot in your armpit!' It worked!"

36

A Rare Diagnosis

Cannon practiced in the same town for more than forty years. However, he began developing a reputation among members of the local medical community very early in his career.

In my second year of practice here in New Albany, I was called for a house call. I went to the patient's home and this kid had a sore throat like I'd never seen before. I took some culture smears of it and took them over to the hospital in Louisville for one of the Sisters to look at—the hospital back then was operated by an order of nuns—so she checked it into the lab and they looked at it.

The next day the Sister called me up all excited and said, "You have a case of diphtheria!"

"Diphtheria?" I replied, "There hasn't been any diphtheria around here for a long, long time."

"Well, you have it," she said simply.

I called the health department and reported the case immediately. We were able to order antitoxin and treat the patient, so he was able to recover from the disease even though a lot of kids didn't make it through diphtheria. And what they did back then was to board up a big plaque across the front of the house that said, "Quarantined."

Because of that sign, practically everyone in town knew something was going on in that house. They could assume there was a serious medical condition. After a couple days, one of the elder doctors in town heard about the diphtheria diagnosis and called me up. "Doctor Cannon," he said, "we haven't had a case of diphtheria here in New Albany for a great many years." I told him I was aware of that. He said, "How come you come to town and all of a sudden you pick up a case? How to you know it's diphtheria?"

I told him, "Well, it looks like it."

"Is that all the proof you have, doctor?" he asked. And I told him that no, as a matter of fact, the Sister at the hospital lab told me what I had.

"Oh," he replied. "You took it to the lab?"

I told him, "Yes I did."

"Oh fine! Why didn't you say so?" He was completely accepting of the whole situation after that.

That was the end of that, but I'm sure glad I took it to the lab. He was ready to rake me over the coals because some junior squirt, just out of medical school, came to town and made an extremely rare diagnosis of diphtheria. You had to simply earn the trust and respect of the older and more experienced doctors.

Yep, glad I got that throat culture!

37

Switching Roles

Many years ago, most emergency rooms essentially closed at night; patients called their doctors if something was wrong, and then the doctors either made house calls or asked the patients to come into their own offices. The emergency rooms were not nearly as busy as they are today, and sometimes they were low on staff. Cannon remembers an experience at his local emergency room that required him to reach beyond his formal education as a physician.

The hospital where I worked was Saint Edward's in Louisville. I would go there to do a surgery or to do rounds on patients later in my career. But in medical school, the emergency room was where I did my training. It was operated by a German order of nuns then, and there was a rather aged nun named Sister Norbetina, who operated the hospital's telephone switchboards.

It was really sparse in there. The emergency room itself wasn't much. It was just a bare room with a table in it and some sutures. There were a few surgical instruments, but that was it. There were no nurses, no attendants, and at night Sister Norbetina was the only one there to help out the doctors or the medical students in training. Back then, the surgeons as well as the general practitioners did their work in their offices. So, it was pretty rare that a patient even came into the emergency room.

If a patient did come, though, they had to come to the emergency room door on the side of the hospital. It was a miniature garage door that came up overhead, and there was another door inside of it that led to the actual emergency room. When somebody pushed the button on the side of the emergency room door, Sister Norbetina would plug in the telephone lines so any calls would go directly to the floor. Then, she could leave her post at the switchboards. She would then go downstairs to the emergency room door. Sometimes I or another one of the doctors would go down with her, and we would hear her yell out the door, "Vell, vat yoo vant?" And the patients had better want what she thought was a very good reason to be there, or she wouldn't open that door.

Once she decided a patient was worthy of being let into the emergency room, we would take care of whatever was needed, but I don't think we got a call to the emergency room more than once a night. It was just not used very much.

There was one night Sister Norbetina got called away and wasn't able to be there to operate the phones. The next night, I found myself in there being taught how to use the switchboard!

38

Four Helpful Sons

Beginning in 1947 Cannon owned and operated his own medical practice. His first office was on the first floor of his home, but when that became a little too close for comfort, he moved the practice next door.

He remembers the rigorous schedule of a solo medical practice and the ways in which having an office so close to home affected his home life.

I was on call twenty-four hours a day. I had office hours during the day and at night, and most days I helped out with surgery at the hospital, too. Sometimes I would have to leave an office full of patients in order to run to the hospital to deliver a baby. If that happened, I would just have to tell my patients to come back to night office hours or the next day. On a typical day, I would finish my surgery by noon and then have time to do my office hours and house calls.

There wasn't anything to mind about working so hard and so many hours. That was just the way it was. You would get weary sometimes. You'd get awfully tired without sleep, but it's just the way the ball bounced.

The one thing I was required to do for my family was to have supper at home every night if I could. I got home for supper most of the time. And most of the time, I was home for lunch, too. That was the nice thing about working so close to home.

I was happier when my office was next door than when it was in my home. It was slightly easier to separate the two lives that way, mentally and physically. I had a patient come in one day with spinal meningitis, and naturally, that meant the whole house could get infected, my kids, too. I had four boys.

Back in those days we also got a whole lot of samples of different kinds of medicine. We could give them to patients in order to help them save money if they were running low. But having all those samples around meant there was always the possibility my boys could get into them. As far as I know, there was never a problem with that—the boys were good about it as far as I know. But, I was sure worried when that spinal meningitis came and walked in.

And, of course, there were a great many cases of measles and mumps and chicken pox coming into the office. It really did worry me, but you just had to get used to it. Luckily we had no problems with any of that.

As the boys got older and my practice moved across the street, my worries about them getting into samples or contracting an illness shifted into awareness that they could help me out from time to time.

I would get them to hold patients down for me if I needed to sew somebody up. My second son came with me once to the hospital because there was a patient with epiglottitis. This condition can cut off the windpipe. My son held the patient down while I got a tube down his throat to help him breathe.

The boys would also come with me on coroner's calls from time to time, too. I was coroner of the county for eighteen years. With that, I averaged about six calls a month. And often I would be babysitting the boys and would get a call, and so we'd all have to drive off on the call. One time, we had to go see a person that had been dead for about a week in his trailer. You could smell the corpse a half-mile away. My boys remember that one; they still talk about it.

I remember one time very well. A mother had brought her son in to my office because he was sick. I decided to give him a shot that would help treat the infection. I had turned around to prepare the shot. But just as I turned back around I saw the boy fly out the door! He'd escaped his mother and just ran out of the office and down the block. But when one of my boys saw this, he ran down the sidewalk and caught the kid. He dragged him back into my office, so I was eventually able to give the kid his shot.

My boys were part of my practice, it seems—a necessary part. I'm not sure what I would have done without them sometimes!

39

"Checking Out"

Raymond Nicholson, MD, was born on May 9, 1930, and was raised in Evansville, Indiana. He graduated from Indiana University in 1952 with a bachelor of science in anatomy and physiology before continuing his education at the IU School of Medicine, graduating in 1955. He subsequently completed internships at the IU Medical Center as well serving with the U.S. Army as a captain.

Nicholson began group practice in 1958. In addition to his private practice, he has had many academic appointments, including assistant clinical professor and clinical professor, both at the IU School of Medicine, and clinical associate professor of pharmacology at Purdue University. He remains active in the medical field, serving as health officer for Vanderburgh County, the director of the Alzheimer Center at Good Samaritan Home in Evansville, Indiana, and the medical director of the Muscular Dystrophy Clinic of Evansville.

Nicholson served as the director of the Saint Mary's Hospital Family Medicine Residency Program in Evansville for many years and received a faculty appointment in the Department of Family Medicine at the IU School of Medicine as a volunteer clinical professor. He

*served as president of the Indiana Academy of Family Physicians from
1990 to 1991.*

*It is sometimes said that while medical specialists may claim expertise in
a certain procedure, disease process, or organ system, the family physician's
area of expertise is people. The ability to read and relate to patients is one of
many attributes that has defined Nicholson's career, and has, on occasion,
helped him save a life.*

Early one evening after a long day in the office that seemed even
longer as the October sun had already set, Nicholson received a frantic
telephone call from one of the residents he was training. "Nick!" the
resident addressed him as most friends and colleagues affectionately
would. "You'd better get over here." The serious tone and rapidity of
speech let Nicholson know that this resident was truly concerned. "This
guy just had a massive heart attack, and now he wants to leave."

The patient was a prominent local businessman, and Nicholson was
aware of his reputation both for creativity in his business and a fiery
temper outside of it. In his calm reply, Nicholson sought not only to
garner more information but also to calm the flustered resident. "Well,
what does the cardiologist have to say?"

The exasperated reply let Nicholson know that this was a situation
that would require a special brand of medical attention: "Well, he's
already fired three of them! They called us in family practice to see
what we could do."

And so Nicholson packed up the last few bits of work he would need
to finish at home and headed over to the main hospital. As he walked
down the corridor to the emergency room, he could already hear some
commotion. Stopping briefly at the nurses' station to verify the patient's
room number, he could see by the expressions on the faces of the nursing staff that the patient was not the only frustrated party. Nicholson
entered the room wearing his famous grin, and introduced himself. The
neatly stacked clothes at the bedside signaled to Nicholson that this
patient was serious about leaving the hospital. The man hesitated only
briefly to exchange pleasantries and then continued the ranting and

raving that had frustrated so many who had proceeded Nick.

"The guy was just ranting and raving about how long he had to wait in the emergency room," Nicholson recalled, "and how the admitting office had treated him; how nobody would give him morphine for the pain, and how he'd had to wait ten minutes for it."

Rather than offer insufficient explanations, or apologize for those who in all likelihood did no wrong, Nicholson simply pulled up a chair, made himself comfortable, and listened. He empathized. "With every complaint I'd just say, 'Gosh, I would hate that,' or 'I'm sorry that happened,'" Nicholson said.

Slowly, Nicholson could see the man's face soften as his anger died down. When the man was again reasonable, the two began to talk and Nicholson, transitioning from listener to physician, explained the man's situation to him. As their discussion drew to a close, the patient shook Nick's hand and said plainly, almost apologetically, "Well, I like you, but damn it, I'm going to leave anyway."

Ever the diplomat, Nicholson responded, "Well that's okay if you want to leave, I just have a couple of pieces of paperwork for you to fill out," reassuring the man that his wishes would be respected.

Nicholson left the room to obtain the necessary paperwork for a patient checking out against medical advice, and returned shortly after filling out his portion. The man was waiting patiently, having not yet changed from his hospital gown. Nicholson first handed the patient a form, which he quickly scanned and signed, acknowledging that he knew he was leaving the hospital against medical advice, and that he was aware of the risks and so on. Once that form was signed the two traded papers, and Nicholson handed him a death certificate that he also filled out in the patient's name. The man again scanned the page quickly, then paused, and read over the sheet of paper again slowly, more carefully. Satisfied that he had read it correctly, he looked up at Nicholson with an expression that evolved from bewilderment to fear. "What is this?" he asked, hoping there was some other explanation.

"Oh, that's just a death certificate," Nick replied calmly, sensing that his point was being received.

"But it has my name on it!"

"I know," said Nicholson, who was now confident that he would be able to get through to the patient, "but if you leave here you're going to die, and so I thought we could just take care of things up front. Let's go ahead and sign this while you can."

That did the trick. The man wisely decided to stay in the hospital and get the necessary treatment that likely saved his life. Nicholson's unique approach had helped to foster not only an effective relationship between doctor and patient, but a friendship as well. "And you know, we became the best of friends," Nicholson happily reported. "He turned out to be one of the nicest guys I ever dealt with."

40

The Sting

It was not unusual in the old days for physicians to accept cash payments from patients, and many times those cash payments were placed directly into the physician's hand. Nicholson remembers a set of house calls that really tested his honesty. His professional integrity saved him a lot of embarrassment and aggravation.

I made house calls on one guy that called me all the time. I could never really pin down what was wrong with him. He had nonspecific abdominal pain, and he always called at night and on weekends.

About three months after I started making house calls on him, all of a sudden an agent from the Internal Revenue Service came busting into my office. He really infuriated me. He was really nasty, and he raised his voice in front of my patients. He wanted to see my books for a particular date. He said, "I don't find this particular man's name in your records."

I asked him what this was all about. He said, "You made a house call on this patient, and I don't see where it was logged in on the date you saw him."

I said, "Well, if I made the house call at night or on a Friday, it probably wasn't logged in until the next work day. Why don't you look a couple days later to see if I put him in at a later date?"

Sure enough the patient was logged in, and he had paid me cash. What was it all about? The IRS wanted to nail me for sticking the money in my pocket and not reporting the income. Apparently, the guy that turns you in to the IRS not only gets half of what he turned you in for, but he gets half of all the money recovered in the audit. So, the patient was just setting me up, assuming that since he always paid cash, I just stuck it in my pocket.

You know, that's exactly what my first partner told me to do when I first started. He said, "If they pay you in cash, just stick it in your pocket, and don't tell anybody about it, and keep it." I never did that. I always reported it.

There's a real lesson here. I could have been nailed really early in my practice. I can see the headline now, "Doctor accused of tax fraud!"

Editor's Note: I recall another story of an Indianapolis general prac-titioner that probably took place in the 1930s or 1940s. This doctor only accepted cash for his services and kept absolutely no records or accounting of his income. No checks were taken, and no bills were ever sent. The story goes that he also never filed a tax return.

One day, IRS agents came knocking at his door and they were not very pleased with him. They threatened audits and prosecution for tax evasion. They had a number of acrimonious meetings with him and demanded his records and payment for many years of unreported income. But there were no records, no proof of his income, and the doctor knew it. The IRS was getting nowhere, and they knew it.

In the end, the IRS told him if he would agree to submit $10,000 they would go away. That's exactly what happened. It is unclear if he ever im-proved his accounting system.

41

A New Disease

Nicholson is known as an excellent diagnostician. But it really helps for a disease to be known to exist before a physician can diagnose it.

Another house call I remember was a woman with an eighteen-year-old son who was Mr. All-American. He was a super athlete in high school and ham radio operator. Everybody knew him. He was killed in a car accident.

Shortly thereafter, she started having headaches. She had one headache after another. My senior partner sent me to her home, even on his call nights, to give her a shot of Demerol for relief. Was it stress? Each time I went, I always would examine her to see if I was missing something.

On about my sixth or seventh trip, her eyes were divergent, and they weren't working together. We brought her to the hospital and worked her up. Remember, we didn't have CTs or MRIs back then. Our main way to image the brain was to drain the cerebrospinal fluid, inject air into the spinal column, and do an air-contrast brain scan. It turned out to be entirely negative. I referred her to IU, and they thought she had a sphenoid sinusitis and treated her with penicillin. We only had three antibiotics back then, and none of them helped. She didn't respond, and finally we thought she probably had a brain tumor but couldn't find anything at all.

We eventually lost track of her and didn't see her for a couple of years. The next time I saw her, she came in and when I looked into the eye, I could see that the optic nerve was entirely dead. It was just a white nerve with total blindness, and she was beginning to have symptoms in the other eye.

About two weeks later, I got a new Cecil textbook of medicine, and it always had a section on, "Diseases Not Previously Described." Listed in there was "temporal arteritis." I looked it up, and it was exactly what this woman had. So, I called her up and had her come in. The textbook recommended the use of prednisone. I put her on that and saved the eye.

She sued me two months later for failure to diagnose her condition when she originally presented. The suit got thrown out, of course. When I first saw her, it was years before the disease was even described.

Can you imagine getting sued for not diagnosing a disease that officially didn't exist yet?

42

You Just Cannot Help Everyone

Herbert Hill, MD, was born in Granite City, Illinois, on July 4, 1937. He attended Wabash College, receiving a bachelor of arts degree in biochemistry in 1959. He graduated from the Indiana University School of Medicine in 1963. Hill completed an internship at Methodist Hospital before entering practice in July 1964. He worked in Indianapolis for many years in two private practices and at M Plan until 2004. Subsequently, he volunteered at the Good News Clinic for low-income and uninsured people until 2012.

Hill also served in the U.S. Army National Guard. Now retired, he resides in Indianapolis with his wife, Gloria.

Doctors learn early in their careers that they can't help all of their patients. And it is especially frustrating when patients can't be helped from themselves.

Family doctors endeavor to treat all of their patients in a support-ive and nonjudgmental manner, regardless of their shortcomings. Some patients are noncompliant with medical recommendations, will not take their medicines as prescribed or obtain diagnostic tests ordered, fail to quit destructive habits such as smoking and excessive drinking, and, despite the

physician's best efforts, cannot seem to follow healthy lifestyles. Still, family
physicians try their best to intervene positively in the lives of their patients
as exemplified by this story told by Hill.

As a family doctor I found myself invested in and responsible for
patients on every level of their health. It wasn't just that somebody
would come in with an injury or a disease and I would fix the problem
and have that be it. No, I knew these people their entire lives in many
instances, and my involvement with their health was very far-reaching. I
went into being a family doctor with the idea of getting to know people
inside and out and helping them with a holistic-type approach to their
health. By that I mean I paid attention to their family dynamic, their
work life, their education, and many other things. All these elements
of a person's life can affect their health in ways that don't necessarily
seem openly apparent.

It's an important thing—and a difficult thing—to strike the
balance between treating patients this way while also not being too
directive in terms of say-
ing, "You have to do this"
or, "You can't do that."
I dealt with the problem
in the case of an older gentleman who was a patient
of mine. He was drinking
himself to death—there is
no plainer way to say it. He
was periodically vomiting
up blood. He had to quit
drinking, he just had to.

But, of course, there was
no way I could make him
quit. There wasn't and there
still isn't any medicine that
he could have taken to help

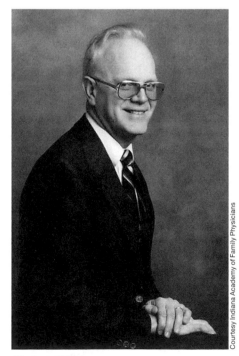

Courtesy Indiana Academy of Family Physicians

Herbert Hill

him quit. I didn't know what to do. I felt I had to figure out a way, no matter what it took, to get my patient to stop drinking.

I asked one of my psychiatrist friends what I should do. I thought maybe he would have something up his sleeve that was a more psychological approach I could use to help my patient. What he said was very instructive to me, and it's a lesson I will never forget. It was blunt, and hearing it stung, but I needed to hear it.

"If they won't go to AA [Alcoholics Anonymous]," he said, "to hell with them."

This basically meant, if a patient doesn't recognize that he has a problem and doesn't want to get help, there's nothing you as a doctor can do.

Treating alcohol abuse and other addictions has been a really difficult thing for me in my career. These sorts of problems don't fall into the usual medical model and are tough to deal with. There's no paradigm for treating them; there is no medicine or guaranteed behavioral treatment program that always works. And if you can't get a patient to even try anything, what can you do?

I would love to be able to say that my patient came around and realized he needed help, and that I was able to direct him towards a treatment program that saved his life, but I can't say that. This patient died from his drinking. I feel sad about that, but I guess some things just come with the territory. Being a family doc isn't easy.

43

Just Let Me Go Home

As Hill experienced, doctors also learn early in their careers that some patients are just difficult and that not all patients will like them. Certainly they find out that they cannot please all patients all of the time!

One of my favorite parts about being a family doctor was building relationships with my patients and getting to know them. Most of the time, the feeling was mutual. But once or twice there were some funny things that happened.

The first office I had was shared with another local doctor, Doctor Brooks. We each had a couple examining rooms and we shared a minor surgical catchall-type room. Our waiting room was also shared. It saw perhaps as many as ten patients at a time.

When Doctor Brooks went on vacation I would sometimes help out and see his patients, especially if there was any sort of emergency. He worked hard and didn't take a lot of vacation, but I do remember one time in particular when he was out for a week or so.

I saw one of Doctor Brooks's patients coming in for a placebo hormone or vitamin shot, and while I hadn't treated her before, I recognized her as Doctor Brooks's patient and welcomed her into the office. I asked her a little bit about how things were going and tried to get to know her a little bit before giving her the shot. I always made it a point to get to know my patients and encouraged them to feel like they could talk to me about anything.

This patient was just a little different.

She said, "I don't want to talk to you! Just give me my shot and let me go home!"

Boy, was she in a bad mood or what? Maybe she didn't like doctors? Or maybe I just didn't have that Doctor Brooks's "magic"? I certainly hoped that I would have better luck with his next patient on my schedule.

Well, I guess what I learned was not every patient wants to be my best friend!

44

Wallpapered Love

Family physicians naturally appreciate the family dynamics that influence their patients' lives and their illnesses. They strive to see their patients in the context of the family and understand how important family love and support is to a patient's well-being. The importance of love is universal and knows no borders. Hill recounts an experience that teaches this important truth.

The most memorable house call I ever made wasn't even in this country. It was in Guatemala. Throughout my career, I frequently went to Central America for mission trips with my church, where I would provide medical care to the folks there who don't have access to the higher levels of care we are used to in America.

Without enough money or options for excellent hospital care, sometimes patients and family members just have to accept the fact that somebody is dying. I learned a lot about love, and about how to practice medicine with love, from going to Central America on these trips.

I remember one patient in particular. She was a young woman who suffered from urinary incontinence. She was a patient of the governmental clinic in Guatemala. The fact of the matter was that she was approaching death. Many times people who have bladder or urinary problems without advanced medical care in a country such as Guatemala will ultimately die from a urinary tract infection.

I tried to help her as best I could, and I tried to figure out what her underlying problem was. I checked her urine, and I recall there was some pus in it. I gave her an antibiotic hoping that would help, but in the end it wasn't enough. I never did understand what caused her basic incontinence. Might it have been repetitive childbirth trauma? I don't know.

As a family doctor you have to understand that you can't save everybody, and that's something you really have to take to heart when you do work in underdeveloped countries. There simply aren't the resources to heal everybody, as much as you wish you could.

I went to visit her on my lunch break one day, and I came into her bedroom for the first time; it nearly brought a tear to my eye. Her family had made a little stool for her to sit on, which was basically a toilet seat for her to be draining into all the time. And while it was a sad, desperate situation, her bedroom was one of the brightest, happiest rooms I saw during my entire visit.

The walls were covered with advertisements from magazines. Bright pictures in every color of the rainbow advertising soft drinks and trips to places all around the world. It was all the family could afford for decoration, but it was just beautiful. They were loving her and taking care of her the best they could as she got ready to die. It was really something to experience.

How fortunate we are to live in America. How much do we simply take for granted?

45

Slippers

Garland Anderson, MD, was born on October 14, 1933, and was raised in Columbia City, Indiana. Before beginning his medical education, Anderson served in the U.S. Navy from 1952 to 1956. He then attended Indiana University for his bachelor of arts degree from the College of Arts and Science, which he received in 1959. He continued his education at the IU School of Medicine, graduating in 1962. He served a rotating internship at Methodist Hospital in Indianapolis.

Anderson entered the practice of family medicine in June 1963. He is still working in Fort Wayne, Indiana, in a group practice. Anderson has a wide scope of practice that includes minor procedures, obstetrics and gynecology, major surgical procedures, anesthesia, and sports medicine. He received a faculty appointment in the Department of Family Medicine at the IU School of Medicine as a volunteer clinical associate professor and was an assistant director of the Fort Wayne Family Practice Residency. In 2005 he was selected as co-Sports Medicine Indiana Physician of the Year.

Anderson and the staff at his private practice felt the desire to help patients and their families with more than medical care. They also attended to their other necessities in life. This desire only amplified during the holiday season.

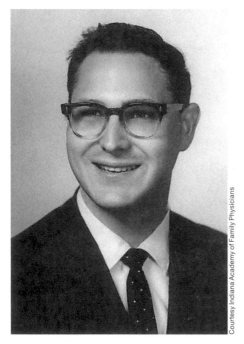

Courtesy Indiana Academy of Family Physicians

Garland Anderson

As part of his office's Thanksgiving and Christmas plans, Anderson and his staff bought groceries for needy patient families. "The people in the office and I would buy groceries and things for our needy families. We'd go to the local grocery store where I got a little deal because I knew the manager. So, we'd get a whole bunch of groceries for two or three families. We'd get some candy and the rest was all good food. We delivered it directly to the door of these people's houses. It was a good experience."

Typically, these were very touching times for the families and for the office. Sometimes it did get amusing. Anderson recalled: "There was one gentleman that we'd treated for a longtime. He was in a nursing home at this point. One of the nurses I'd had for a longtime, JoAnn, asked him what he would like for Christmas. He told her he would love a new pair of house slippers.

"So, she goes out and buys them. She takes them over to him at the nursing home and in his room he has loads of house slippers, brand new ones, lying all around. Unfortunately, the man had Alzheimer's, and it was getting worse. The nurse said that he must've told everyone to get him house slippers."

46

Holding a Hand

With close to fifty years as a family physician, Anderson cared for many patients through all of life's stages over many years. So naturally, Anderson became very close and extraordinarily fond of some of his patients. A number of their stories still strike a soft spot for him today. After all, it is the face-to-face, personal, patient care that he feels makes family medicine different from other specialties.

One of those stories was about an eighty-two-year-old woman. "She was a Lutheran minister's wife," Anderson recalled. "Her son was a surgeon in North Carolina. She had been a patient of mine for a very long time. She came in very fatigued and sick one day. To make a long story short, four to six months later she passed away. She died of leukemia.

"Before she died, she was in our hospice section of the hospital for her end-of-life care. She called my nurse because she didn't think I knew she was there. So, I went to visit her and told her that, indeed, I had already known that she was there. I had visited her previously but did not wake her up. The nurse was supposed to tell her that I had come.

"She turned to me and put out her hand. I held it. Not much was said for some time. Then she said, 'I just want to thank you, doctor.' It was the only reason she wanted me to visit her. She merely wanted to have the opportunity to thank me.

"Well, all it takes is a thank you. Some of these types of memories makes me a bit teary eyed still."

47

The Old Days

James Asher, MD, was raised in New Augusta, Indiana. He began his undergraduate work at Purdue University. He later received his bachelor of science degree from Indiana University, as well as his medical degree from the IU School of Medicine in 1942. Asher completed an internship at Methodist Hospital in Indianapolis in 1943 before entering private practice in New Augusta (later incorporated into the City of Indianapolis).

Asher worked with his father, Ernest Asher, MD, for more than twenty years. In 1997, after fifty-three years of practice, Doctor Jim, as he was affectionately known, retired from medicine. Although retired, he continued to volunteer throughout Indianapolis in clinics for the homeless with a group called Volunteers in Medicine. Asher died on May 14, 2007.

Asher provided the author with a potpourri of quips, memories, and wisdom. Taken together, you can get a feel for the essence of his career and a flavor of how family medicine was practiced a half century ago.

You really come to love your patients. I miss some of them still since I retired. The relationships were so important. It wasn't work.

I loved it. I had a number of patients that had been my father's. We were in practice for twenty years together in the same office. I learned a great deal from him. When my dad started practicing he used a horse and buggy.

My dad made an agreement with one of his patients. This blacksmith took care of his horse, and my dad took care of his family. Eventually the car came along, and they modified the deal. This fellow would now take care of my car, and I would take care of his family. I was still taking care of the daughter until 1987, when she died. When I say "take care," I mean free of charge.

We went to the store yesterday and bumped into a lady that I had taken care of for many years. Actually, I delivered their first child in 1946, and I took care of the family until I retired. We are always bumping into somebody that I took care of.

I always tried to go to my patients' funerals or visitations. We had a niece that visited from Virginia. We had to go to the funeral home and I told her, "Tammy, they keep this parking place reserved for me." They actually did.

She said, "I thought you were supposed to cure them, not kill them."

House calls were a daily routine for me. I remember that one day I made twenty calls. And you know, they always didn't turn out to be for a medical problem!

I once made a call on a German lady who had requested a house call. When I got there she said, "Doctor, I'm not sick. I've just got some new music, and I want you to polka with me." So, we danced a couple of polkas. She paid me, and I went on my way.

There was another patient I had down in an area that flooded often. This lady bought a player piano, and any time I made a house call there, I had to sit down on the bench with her while she played the "chipmunks," which she was very fond of. She had an arrangement with the Baldwin Music Company that if a flood was coming, they would come and get her player piano out of there before it could get wet.

When I was actively practicing OB we would have about one delivery per week. I would provide prenatal care, do the delivery, and then a six-week exam. I had this mother with a baby out of wedlock. The mother of the pregnant girl had brought her into the office. She was in active labor, and I told them we needed to get her to the hospital. I was helping her to the car and she said, "I can't wait." She delivered on the front porch of the office.

When I was a medical student I used to do "outdoor OB" at the City General Hospital. The patient would call the hospital, and the junior and senior medical students would grab their bag of "tools," go to the home to deliver, and then maybe go back for several days for postpartum care. My mother would not let me in the house when I was on-call for OB at City Hospital. I had to change clothes and shower in the garage, empty my suitcase and spray it, so I wouldn't bring any vermin into the house. She was very sincere about that.

One Sunday before we were married, my future wife was here. We were going out for lunch, and she was supposed to leave for Bloomington at 5:00 p.m. I had to go to a home delivery, and it was July, and it was blazing hot. She took the newspaper with her and locked the doors of the car (we were in a bad neighborhood). I told her it wouldn't take long. I was still in there at 7:00 p.m. and her bus was long gone. She spent many hours over the years waiting for me. She learned to keep books in the car and activities for the kids to do. She's been very patient with me over the years.

I think antibiotics were probably the biggest thing that changed medicine during my career. I saw the introduction of all of that. Some would wear out, but there was always another one in the pipeline. When penicillin first came out, everybody wanted it for anything that came up from a sneeze to an operation. A relative of my wife developed strep throat and died. The day after she died they released sulfa. It's easy to take antibiotics and immunizations and all our medical advancements for granted. We live in a wonderful time.

Many of the people we hear from now say that they don't like the doctor they have today. They say it's not like it was when they came to me. I think I was good about reassuring people. I always gave my patients whatever amount of time they needed. I always tried to remember things about my patients and their families. We would cut out clippings about their family and keep it in their file. When they came for the next call, we had a little piece of something nice to talk with them about. We really developed relationships with our patients. Everybody knew everybody.

48

Big Ears

Harry Wolf, MD, was born on December 29, 1931, and spent his childhood in Indianapolis, Indiana. He studied business at Indiana University for his undergraduate degree, graduating in 1953. He then continued at the IU School of Medicine, receiving his medical degree in 1966. Additionally, Wolf served in the U.S. Army for two years.

Wolf began practicing in Indianapolis in 1966, first as a solo physician but then in group practice. His career as a family doctor included obstetrics and inpatient hospital work. After selling his practice to Saint Vincent Hospital, Wolf began teaching in the hospital's family medicine residency program. He retired from practice in 2003. He received a faculty appointment in the Department of Family Medicine at the IU School of Medicine as a volunteer clinical assistant professor.

Wolf was asked what the best part of being a family doctor was:

Oh, I guess, making people feel better, which is not the same thing as curing their disease. You can cure their disease and make them feel lousy, or sometimes you can make them feel good and not cure their

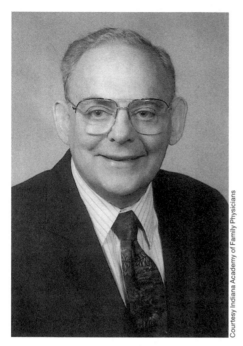

Courtesy Indiana Academy of Family Physicians

Harry Wolf

disease. So, you want to strive to do both, but they are separate. Even if you can't cure their disease, you can usually find some way to make them feel better.

One lady told me once that if she were going to draw a picture of me, she would draw a great big ear. I do have pretty big ears. But she told me that I always listened to what she had to say, and I always tried to keep that in mind. One of the biggest complaints I got from patients about other doctors was that "He always rushed me through or he never listened to me; or his mind was always on something else." You have to be careful not to get into that groove. If you are a family physician you have to listen to the patient attentively, and let the patient do some talking.

I had a professor once that said, "If you listen to the patient closely, they will tell you what is wrong with them."

I was never that concerned with being the "great God doctor." When I went on vacations, I wouldn't sign in as "Doctor Wolf" or anything. Sometimes doctors complain about the hard work. My father was in the automobile business, and I always said that I thought it was harder work selling cars than it was being a doctor.

49

Those Calls in the Middle of the Night

Doctors do get those late-night phone calls from patients. Physicians will tell you the later the phone call, if not from the emergency room, the greater the chance the caller is an odd person with a strange complaint.

The reader may be familiar with the story of the doctor who was awakened by a phone call from a patient in the middle of the night. The woman called to let the doctor know that she could not sleep. The doctor's response: "Now we both can't sleep!"

Wolf's story is just about the same situation:

I remember once, a physician friend of mine went to the Rose Bowl the year Indiana University went. He asked me to take calls for him while he was gone. I got a call at 2:00 a.m. It was a young person's voice, and she said, "Well, my mother asked me to call and see if you know why she is so tired all the time."

I didn't say it, but I thought, "Maybe you should ask her if she's fatigued because she's up at 2:00 a.m. wondering why she is so fatigued!"

50

House Calls

House calls were, of course, an expected and routine part of Wolf's family practice career. He reminisces about house calls early in his practice:

We used to make house calls for ten dollars. I made about one house call per day during the first year or two of practice.

I stopped making house calls because of the increase in the number of fully staffed emergency rooms. When I started practice, when somebody called with chest pain, I would grab my bag and my portable EKG machine and go to the patient's home. If they were having a heart attack, I would have to call the ambulance. Within three years or so of when I started practicing, house calls went by the wayside because the hospitals were hiring full-time staff for their ERs. We could then send the patients to the hospital directly to be evaluated and hospitalized if needed. I continued doing house calls on older people that couldn't get out of the house. And there weren't nursing homes on every corner like there are now. Lots of the bedfast old folks were staying in the home and could not get to the doctor.

I remember the last day in my practice. I got a call from the wife of a patient of mine, and he was very sick. He had a cough and I could hear him in the background. It would have been hard for him to get out of bed to come in, and I didn't think he really needed the ER. So, I stopped by the home to see him, and I thought he had pneumonia but didn't need to be hospitalized. So, I prescribed some antibiotics and gave him a shot of something. House calls were a real service for patients, especially for those who otherwise may not have received the care they needed for one reason or another. I never minded doing them when patients really needed me to come out, even on the last day of my practice.

I once did a house call on a lady who was referred to me by the Medical Society Exchange because she didn't have a physician. It was an apartment complex, and I went to her apartment and examined her. I needed to use a telephone. She had a daughter living with her in the home, but they had no telephone.

So, I went down the hall and there was a lady standing outside the door of her apartment and I said, "I'm a doctor, could I borrow your telephone?" She started screaming and shrieking. I turned and went back to the apartment and closed the door. I guess she didn't like doctors. I didn't try that ever again!

51

From the Tropics to the Hoosier State

David Hadley, MD, was born on January 10, 1928, and graduated from Friends Boarding School in Barnesville, Ohio, in 1945. He attended Guilford College in Greensboro, North Carolina, receiving his bachelor of science degree in chemistry. He graduated in 1952 from the University of Pennsylvania School of Medicine in Philadelphia. Hadley served an internship at Charity Hospital in New Orleans, Louisiana, where he also served a year of an internal medicine residency. He then served as a medical officer in the U.S. Navy from 1954 to 1956.

After being in solo family practice for two years in Tellico Plains, Tennessee, Hadley served eight years as a missionary physician at Kaimosi Hospital, Kenya. While on two different furloughs, he took two years of surgical residency at Truesdale Hospital, now Union Hospital, in Fall River, Massachusetts, and later another two-year surgical residency at Miami Valley Hospital, Dayton, Ohio.

In 1971 Hadley entered into private practice in Plainfield and Danville, Indiana. He retired from private practice in 2002. He continues to work as the Hendricks County Health Officer. He has received a number of awards, including the Indiana Academy of Family Physicians' Lester

Bibler Award in 1995 for his outstanding contributions to the specialty of family medicine in Indiana.

Hadley had a desire to practice tropical medicine, but he still ended up in Indiana. He went to western Kenya for four years doing charity work. He worked with an English doctor for two of those years; it was a general practice performing anything that the village needed.

In Kenya, a stay in the hospital cost the equivalent of twenty-eight cents. "Of course, we had a lot of people that couldn't even afford that," he said. "We'd have people bring in bananas or chicken, sometimes a live chicken, to pay their bill. Of course, when you think about it, in rural America it also wasn't unusual for patients to bring their family doctors similar things from their farms and fields or gardens."

As one would expect, the technology available in Kenya was considerably less than in America. Hadley mentions that after four years in Africa, it was difficult getting used to the medical amenities in the United States. He returned to the states and took a couple years of surgery training beginning in 1963 in southeast Massachusetts before returning to Africa for another four years.

"We saw a lot of surgery and did a lot of caesareans," he said. "We saw a lot of tropical diseases. Once, we opened up a woman for a bowel obstruction and found that the cause was that her small and large intestines were just filled with worms. So we had to remove all the worms and stitched her back up. She recovered okay. We didn't suspect that worms were causing the obstruction before the surgery. It was quite a shock, as you would imagine.

"Another time, we had this child who was just two to three years old brought to the hospital by her father. The child had these lesions which looked like multiple bites on the back. I wasn't sure what it was, but when you pressed them, out would pop a worm. When the child saw it, she was fit to be tied.

"I attempted some surgeries which were quite successful, but some were not. I recall one baby who had a depressed skull fracture. We had a nurse anesthetist who put the baby to sleep, and I made an incision

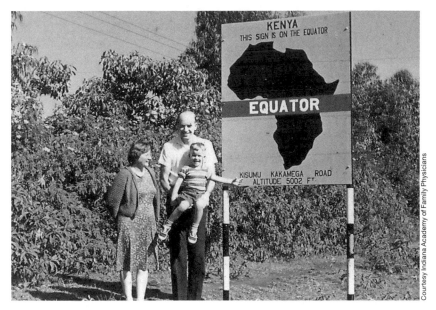

David Hadley and family.

and popped the skull back out in that place. The Africans were quite impressed by that even though it was not that difficult.

"I remember my first C-section. In making one of the incisions, I wasn't careful enough, and I cut off the tip of the little finger of the baby. Of course, here in the United States that would have resulted in a malpractice suit. But there, the family accepted this; they were just grateful that she was alive. About six or seven years later during my second term there, they brought her back and asked if I remembered her. They held up her hand with the tip of her finger gone. We all had a good laugh about it."

In spite of his training as a surgeon, Hadley realized that he was called for family medicine. In 1971 he came to Plainfield and practiced until 2002. He continues to serve as the county health officer, a position commonly held by family doctors in rural areas.

"Back in those days we made quite a few house calls, but I didn't do any home deliveries in Hendricks County," Hadley recalled. "We did have an African American population in Plainfield at the time, and I recall one old black gentleman who was in his nineties. He told about his uncle and how he escaped from the South during slavery by hiding in the bottom of a wagon covered with hay. He enthralled me with all his stories when I made house calls to him. I think I benefited from him more than he did from me.

Before finishing his career in Indiana, Hadley practiced in rural eastern Tennessee. There he did a lot of home deliveries in the mountains, where the roads were unpaved and extremely rough. There was a mountain nursing service that would tide patients over until they could get to the hospital some twenty miles away in Sweetwater. He describes a few home deliveries of pregnant women: "We'd just have them on their bed. We'd put a board, or something, under the bed to make the mattress more firm. We'd have them lying crosswise and then just put their legs up and deliver the baby right there. We'd use open-drop ether which my wife administered. You know, it's pretty safe. Except for the open fire in the next room!"

52

Not the Brightest Nurse

Charles McClary, MD, was born on April 5, 1936, and was raised in Evansville, Indiana. He attended Vanderbilt University for his undergraduate studies before studying medicine at the Indiana University School of Medicine, graduating in 1960. He completed an internship at Marion County General Hospital in Indianapolis.

McClary entered practice in 1961, working with the U.S. Navy until 1963, when he began working in Bloomington, Indiana, in private practice. He worked in a partnership until his retirement in 2003. He received a faculty appointment at the Indiana University School of Medicine Department of Family Medicine as a volunteer clinical assistant professor.

McClary knew full well that some things were just different years ago. The way people interacted with one another was different. And, as history has shown us, the way people interacted with those who were different from them was also, well, different. McClary always strived to be a great family doctor to all of his patients, and he made every effort to treat them all equally. Unfortunately, sometimes he had to compensate for the rest of his staff, who just were not as worldly as he was. He remembers when he had to handle a situation created by one of his nurses:

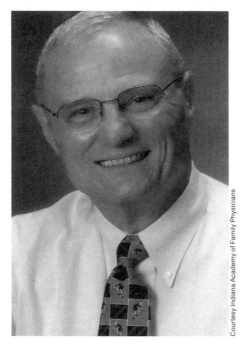

Courtesy Indiana Academy of Family Physicians

Charles McClary

I remember an incident from when I was in my office on Third Street in Bloomington. We had a patient come in who was an African American man. He was an ROTC officer, a really upstanding guy, and he came in to see me for a strep throat.

Well, back in those days you gave someone with strep throat a shot of penicillin and ten days worth of pills. Penicillin was about all we had, so we used it for most problems including strep throat. All that had to be administered to this young man was a shot of penicillin. It was a very simple procedure.

Since we had administered penicillin shots so many times at my office, I sometimes had my nurses handle that kind of thing. I had a couple nurses working for me then. The one who was assigned to give this ROTC officer a shot was a registered nurse who, God help her, was actually dumb as a brick. I had to let her go later, but it turned out she was able to do some damage before that time came.

I told her to give this patient a shot of penicillin and pills for his strep throat, and then I went off to attend to two or three other patients who were in for various things.

After about ten or twenty minutes, the nurse comes and finds me. I excuse myself from the patient I'm with, and we're standing out in the hallway and she is holding an alcohol swab that's all brown.

She said to me, "Doc, I need your help. I don't know what to do. I can't get this guy clean enough to give him a shot!"

I'd forgotten who the patient was, so I go back with her to

examining room number five where this patient is sitting. I go back there, and there's this guy sitting on the operating table with a big grin on his face. He says to me, "Doc, call her off! She's about to rub a hole in me!" Oh boy, this patient knew he had a real lamebrain working on him. Of course, this nurse was rubbing and rubbing, and she was rubbing the pigment right off his arm! I sighed and said, "Go ahead give him the shot." It was a different time back then.

53

Take One Practical Joke, Twice a Day

McClary delivered babies, bandaged scrapes and cuts, and diagnosed diseases, sometimes serious ones. But he is quick to tell you that the relationships he had with his patients were often the most rewarding part of his job. It made his career truly worthwhile.

A family practice doctor sees many characters come in and out of his office doors, and they all bring something different to the table. Some are sweet, some are talkative, some are funny, and some are downright ornery. But a family doctor loves nothing if not people, and if he's lucky, he'll open his heart enough to let his patients come in and make him smile or laugh, or shake his head in wonder.

Back before the days of rapid-fire doctor visits, before emergency care centers were as popular as they are now, before insurance companies required doctors to document their every step—before all that, there was more time to spend with patients. And how much fun that could be. McClary provides an example:

I had this patient, Andy, who was one hundred years old. He was a retired engineer, and anyone who knows engineers knows that they are a very specific breed of person. They're very literal. They want proof, they think logically, and they think in terms of, "it is what it is." There isn't much middle ground, much gray, for engineers. And Andy, he was a true engineer type. I'll never forget him. His goal was simple—to live to one hundred. And he made it to one hundred. Even at one hundred years old, he still drove to the office himself.

He loved to tease me, give me hell. He always wanted to have a little fun no matter what he was sick with. So one day, he's in the office, and I walk into the examining room and say, "Andy, how are you doing?"

"Doc," he says, "I'm great," and he pulls a vial of medicine out of his pocket. "But doc, I've just got one problem. I can't take your medicine the way it says here."

"What do you mean? What's the problem?" I asked him.

"Well, look here. It says you take one pill twice a day. I can take the pill the first time, but how do I get it back to take the second time? Do I put a string on it and pull it back out or what?" And he gives me this look like, "Okay big boy, what are you gonna do with that?"

It was one of those things that you could tell he'd been sitting at home in his easy chair just bringing himself to tears thinking about how he was going to put one over on the doc. He knew I'd get as big a kick out of it as he did, probably!

So, I looked at him very seriously and patted him on the back. I told him that I was going to take care of it and that he shouldn't worry. I was very sorry for the mistake. What I did next was something that I expected to hear from the pharmacist about, because I decided to play Andy's own game with him!

So what did I do? Well, I rewrote every last one of his prescriptions to say, "Take one pill in the morning, then take a different pill in the afternoon!" I sent it off to the pharmacy, so the next time he got his prescription he'd know that I was up for a little joke just as much as he was!

54

Oh, the Places You'll Go and Still Be Recognized!

One thing any family doctor will tell you is that, even when you retire, you never stop being a family doctor. Even if you are no longer practicing, your patients will always remember you as their doc. Whether they are asking you about their back pain in the checkout line at the grocery store, or catching you up about their grandchildren at the funeral of a beloved neighbor, your patients always keep a special place for you in their hearts and prayers.

Often this kind of recognition is limited to the town in which the doctor practiced, but not always. Sometimes, your career will follow you far and wide—even across oceans. McClary remembers being recognized, during his retirement, in the most unlikely of places:

Since I retired, my wife and I have been traveling a lot. One time, we were in a little hotel in Aix en Provence in the south of France. We went there because we felt it would be beautiful and a real getaway, you know? We wanted to travel somewhere special together, away from Indiana, where we could just kind of escape and get lost amongst the locals. Well, we were waiting to get on an elevator at our hotel and you'll never guess what we saw.

Here's this young man standing there holding his suitcase and wearing an Indianapolis Motor Speedway t-shirt! My wife Judy looked at his t-shirt and said, "You must be from Indiana."

"Well, yes I am," he says. "I'm living in Indianapolis right now, but I grew up in Bloomington."

"Well, what a small world. We live in Bloomington," Judy says.

We asked him where he grew up in Bloomington, and it turns out it was the very next street over from us! The world was getting smaller by the minute.

The world quickly got even smaller. Turns out I'd delivered him and taken care of him until he went away to college. What a wonderful reunion and what fun reminiscing about his family and our doctor's visits together. It was rewarding to see that he had grown into a nice young man.

55

An Unexpected Visit

McClary recalls a blizzard many years ago that made it difficult for patients to see their doctors. Thank goodness for strong relationships between them. It is one of the hallmarks of family medicine.

There was a huge blizzard in town that basically shut all the businesses down. It led people to stay inside and kind of just wait it out. Well, the next day after the first big snow of that blizzard, I wanted to get to my office, which was just down at College Mall, pretty close to where I lived with my wife and kids. At the time, I had some cross-country skis. So, I strapped them on tight, and it wasn't really all that difficult for me to just ski over there!

I thought I'd answer the phones and help people as I could over the phone. So that's what I was doing, just answering the phones and talking to my patients that way. I got a couple of phone calls, and the callers were pretty surprised the doc was in! I told them there's no way I'd have been able to make it over without my cross-country skis! Everyone who called had a pretty good laugh about that.

Now, in family practice at that time, you found that you had some certain patients who were just sturdy folks. They're the kind of people that keep to their word, no matter what. Farmers are like that, and so were the stone quarry workers in Bloomington. This guy was one of these tough old guys who worked in the stone quarries. And they're just tough. They're a tough breed. They just take care of business.

On the day of the big blizzard, I'd been at the office a couple hours, and at about 10:30 a.m. the front door opens, and I hear this stomping in the waiting room. I thought, well that just simply couldn't be. Could it? How could anyone make it here? Literally all the roads in town were shut down.

So I go out expecting, I guess, to see someone with a snowplow or some big strong young guy. Heck, maybe even a cop. It would have taken something serious to get someone out here in this weather!

Well, here's this eighty-year-old patient of mine. A stone quarry worker named John who lived in Smithville, outside of Bloomington. "Good grief John," I said, "What are you doing here?"

I thought somebody was having a heart attack or something. What on earth would have brought someone out here in this weather, from Smithville no less?

"Well doc, today's my appointment. I came in to have my emphysema checked."

I said, "My god, how'd you get here?"

"Well it was tough. I was the first car out of town." He looked out the window at his rusty old beat up pickup truck. "My appointment's at 10 o'clock," he said, "and by god, I'm gonna show up! Sorry I'm late, doc."

You know, they just don't make 'em that tough anymore.

56

It's All in the Family

Family doctors in small-town Indiana in the 1950s and 1960s were often responsible for taking care of the entire community. In some towns, there were only a few or even just one doctor for the whole community. Inevitably, this resulted in the doctor knowing almost everyone in town.

However, that doesn't mean the doctor always knew who in town might be related to one another. McClary remembers:

I spent about twenty years doing obstetrics. After the end of that time, I had delivered a couple thousand babies. And I'll never forget one night that I got called over for a delivery at the hospital at about three o'clock in the morning.

This was back when the father had to wait in the waiting room while the baby was delivered. The father would wait for the doctor to come out and tell him whether it was a boy or a girl. I think you know the scene. So I delivered the baby, and I was going out to tell the father. I knew the hard part was over, and I really wanted to get home and get some sleep. Keep in mind it was three in the morning at that point! And I had to go to my regular office hours in the morning.

Well, I walked into the waiting room and the father stood up, but then also maybe fifteen other people stood up too, and they all came toward me. I'll tell you what, I was pretty sleepy at that point, and it was just like one of these horror movies! All these bodies were coming toward me like they were zombies getting ready to swallow me up or something!

I thought, "Holy smokes, what's going on?" I took a closer look, and it turned out they were all patients of mine. Every last one. And I just didn't know what to make of it. "My god," I thought, "are they all sick? What's going on?"

Well, it turns out they were all relatives of this lady who had had a baby—all fifteen of them—and they'd all showed up at the hospital to hear about the baby. That's a small town for you!

57

Strong-Arming Your Patients

Family practice doctors could sometimes be found just helping people any way they could. They had solid relationships with their patients. There was an unspoken understanding that patients could just call you for anything they needed help with. "Call the doc. He'll help." McClary remembers one time his help was needed in a very nontraditional way:

The wife of this guy, a patient of mine, called me and said, "Bill's under the house and I can't get him out! Come help!" Well, I knew the wife because she was a nurse at the hospital, so I knew she wasn't a nutcase. But she was pretty frantic on the phone and didn't explain much. I went over there to help, of course, I had to go. But I didn't know exactly what was going on. I didn't know what to expect, I just went over there rather blindly.

So, I go to their house and there's John in the crawlspace underneath the house. He hurt his back and he couldn't get himself out. Now, she couldn't pull him out because his back was completely out; she wasn't strong enough to haul out all that weight of his! Turns out he'd gone under there to fix a pipe.

So, what could I do? I crawled in the crawl space and dragged him out. He was screaming and hollering all the way about his back and that I was killing him or something.

Seems to me like they should've called a strong friend of theirs, or a tow truck—hah! But no, I was happy to help. That was part of the job. Some of the "work" you did wasn't stuff you learned in medical school. You just helped out in your community, and your patients knew they could call on you for anything.

I'm just glad I'd done my pushups that week!

58

Listening

It is an undeniable fact that there were substantially fewer medicines and treatments to offer patients in the mid-twentieth century. This may seem like an unfortunate fact of the times, but that was not necessarily relevant in many cases. Doctors back then sometimes had to be a little more inventive when diagnosing and treating their patients. Many physicians found that, despite all the training they received during medical school, their patients were not always interested in the knowledge in their brains or the steadiness of their hands. No, sometimes all patients wanted from their doctor was someone to listen. McClary well remembers the time he learned this very valuable lesson:

Late one afternoon, I was finished with my workday. It was early evening, and I was in my office doing the charts for the day. I was dictating the charts to one of the nurses. A secretary comes back and says, "Mrs. Smith is here—she says she's just got to see you."

I said, "OK."

Back then doctors didn't really keep strict "work hours" the way they do now. You were responsible for your patients, and you took care of them. And if they needed extra attention or extra time, that was part of it.

I put down the charts—I would come back to them later, whenever—and walked into the examining room. I said, "Sally what's the trouble?" As soon as she started to talk, it was like floodgates had opened. She just went on and on and on. She talked and talked and talked. And I couldn't get a single word in. And you know that's okay. But I didn't know that then.

This was a difficult thing for me to experience as a doctor because I was there with my patient—a person I am supposed to help, and she's just letting out this avalanche of problem after problem. None of the problems she was telling me about was anything I knew how to fix or help with. In fact, I didn't even know who to send her to for help.

"Doctor, my daughter is pregnant."

"Doctor, my boyfriend is in prison."

"Doctor, I don't know what to do!"

It was just one horrible thing after the other. They were just disasters. And I'm sitting there thinking, "My god, there's nothing I can do about this." I didn't know where to send her or what to do about it all. I was getting really worried. Was she expecting me to be able to fix these issues with her family? Did she think I would have the answers she'd been looking for? I was seriously beginning to doubt myself as a family doctor. I was supposed to help people, but I just didn't know how to help this woman.

Well, after about twenty minutes, she lets out a big sigh and she looks directly at me. I start to open my mouth to tell her how sorry I was and that I had to let her down—I couldn't help. But before I could get any of that out, she rose from her seat and said, "Well thanks a lot, I feel a lot better!" Then she got up and walked out. I never said a word the whole time!

It became clear to me then that she just wanted to vent. She wanted somebody to hear her story. And it's interesting how much help that is to patients, and how much good that does. You don't really know that until you learn it for yourself. I'm worried about young doctors. When are they going to give themselves a chance to learn that lesson?

For me, it was possibly the very most important lesson I learned in all my years as a doc.

59

Obstetrical Surprises

Wallace "Bill" Adye, MD, was born on December 16, 1928, and was raised in Spencer County, Indiana. He began his studies for his bachelor of science degree at Evansville College before moving to Indiana University, graduating in 1949. Adye was given an appointment to West Point Military Academy but declined it to enter medical school. He received his medical degree from IU in 1953.

Adye entered family medicine in 1954, but also served as a captain in the U.S. Air Force. After he returned, he and his partner settled in Evansville, Indiana, where they alternated night calls and office hours. He delivered up to a hundred babies per year at three different Evansville hospitals before he stopped obstetrics work. Additionally, the partners performed minor surgery, with one performing the surgery and the other giving anesthesia.

A particularly proud moment for Adye was when he delivered a set of triplets with only the help of one nurse. He has served as the president of the Indiana Academy of Family Physicians (1991 to 1992), president of Deaconess Hospital in Evansville, and president of the Vanderburgh County Medical Society. Adye received a faculty appointment in the Department of Family Medicine at the IU School of Medicine as a volunteer clinical *associate professor and was the director of the Deaconess Family Medicine Residency Program for many years. Adye and his wife Alice Jayne resided in Evansville. Adye died on May 23, 2013.*

Family physicians could have some really interesting experiences doing obstetrics. It comes with the territory. Usually everything goes as expected; it's a natural process we usually just help along. But surprises do occur while delivering babies, especially at a time when the standards of care were much looser and not as exacting. It was a time when the technology was less advanced and available, and when family doctors handled situations that today would be routinely referred to obstetricians. Adye reminisces about two such cases:

My partner and I both delivered babies, and it was not uncommon for us to deliver each other's patients when covering for one another on call. Sometime during the prenatal period we would see each other's patients, so the patients would be familiar and more comfortable with both of us.

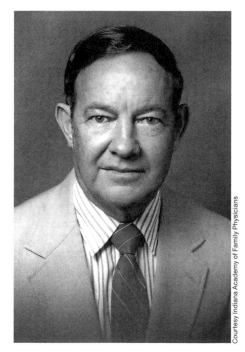

Courtesy Indiana Academy of Family Physicians

One night I went in to deliver a baby, and there was a family doc doing anesthesia. He used open-drop ether most of the time. I had met this patient, but I didn't really know much about her; my partner hadn't told me anything in particular about her. So, she went through labor, and I delivered a little girl. Nothing unusual.

The anesthetist would sometimes help with the delivery as there were just the two of us. He said to me, "Doc, I think there is another

Wallace "Bill" Adye

one in there." So, I went in and ruptured another bag of water and delivered a twin. Twins were a little unusual but no huge deal, really. I was working with the two babies and he said, "Doc, I think you got another one." So, I delivered triplets that night with no forewarning. Now that's really unusual.

You know, if you have triplets nowadays, you would have three pediatricians and two obstetricians and a room full of nurses. So, the two of us took care of the triplets and the mother, and they all did fine. I got cards and pictures of them until they were in about fifth or sixth grade.

I went to the waiting room and said to the father, "I have some news, and I don't know if it is good news or bad news, but you now have three new little girls."

"You've got to be kidding me doc!"

"No, I'm not. Congratulations!"

Terrified, he said, "Goddamn doc, I've got three girls at home."

You know, when you deliver twins, let alone triplets, bad things can happen. I was fortunate that everything turned out well with a healthy mother and three babies. Another time on a Thanksgiving Day things didn't turn out so well, unfortunately.

The nurses called and told me I needed to check this laboring patient. I said, "Why do I have to come in to check her? You do this all the time, and I just deliver four to five times a month. You know more about it than I do!"

They said, "No, you've got to come in, doctor. We did a vaginal check and can't figure out what part of the baby is presenting." So, I went over there and did the pelvic exam and couldn't tell what the hell I was feeling. I thought I had better get some help. This was really strange.

I called the obstetrician, and he wasn't there. I finally got his partner, and he was really sarcastic and said, "Let me get this straight. As long as you've been delivering babies, you can't tell on exam what the baby's presentation is?"

I was pretty frustrated and said, "No, why don't you just come on out here and take a look yourself." In the interim, I went ahead and got an X-ray which told me exactly what was going on. But I wasn't about to tell him. So when he came, he examined her and didn't know what was going on either! He needed to be humbled a little, so I let him wonder for a while, and then I told him. What we had was Siamese twins and we were feeling where their heads had joined together, and it wasn't a complete union. So, we had to do a C-section to get them out. They passed away, of course. Doing obstetrics wasn't always a happy time.

60

Delivering Babies

Paul Siebenmorgen, MD, was born on September 16, 1920, in Terre Haute, Indiana. After receiving his bachelor of science in education from Indiana State Teacher's College in 1941, he attended the Indiana University School of Medicine, graduating in 1944.

Siebenmorgen completed an internship at Methodist Hospital in Indianapolis in 1945 and served as a captain in the U.S. Army Medical Corps during World War II.

In 1947 Siebenmorgen began practice in Terre Haute. In addition to his practice, he was greatly involved in organized medicine, including the Indiana Academy of Family Physicians and the Indiana State Medical Association. His positions included chairmanship of the Indiana State Medical delegation to the American Medical Association in 1986 and serving as president of the Indiana Academy of Family Physicians from 1980 to 1981. Locally, he was active with the Terre Haute Medical Education Foundation and many other organizations.

Siebenmorgen, one of Indiana's most beloved and respected family doctors, died on August 12, 2009.

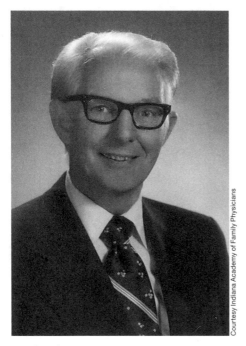

Courtesy Indiana Academy of Family Physicians

Paul Siebenmorgen

Driving was a stressor for Siebenmorgen. "Anytime I was in the car, going places or to a make a house call, it was a waste of time," the eighty-five-year-old physician recalled. "My wife always complained that I was pushing to get where I was going. Well, that was the way I had to be for so long. It's still hard to keep it down to the speed limit."

It wasn't the act of driving that bothered him; it was the lack of being able to help someone who needed him. This unselfish devotion to his patients was a hallmark of this family doctor for fifty-three years. "Sitting in the car is a waste of time," he declared.

His desire to help anyone in need was all he ever knew. The son of a physician, "Doctor Paul," as his patients called him, could recite his father's credo typed on a paper under the glass blotter on his desk: "We're not on this earth to make a living, but to make a life worth living." This motto followed him throughout his days of medical school and internships in the U.S. Army during World War II. Within days after returning to Terre Haute, Siebenmorgen was called into action. It was around Christmas 1946.

"My dad was supposed to deliver a baby but he had the flu. He was feeling so terrible that right in the middle of everything, he had to go out and sit in a chair, and I delivered the baby," he said. It was to be the first of more than five thousand births that Siebenmorgen performed.

"That was the fun part of practicing medicine," he said of delivering so many babies. "It's the joy of bringing in a new life, everybody in the family getting excited, calling Grandma on the phone. You know, all that kind of stuff."

In the mid-twentieth century home births were still common. Movies, books, and even television are full of home-birth references. The doctor would command a washbasin full of hot water and old sheets would be torn into strips. In addition to the economies of home births, Siebenmorgen said there were added advantages. The mother had a lower risk of infection because she was well acquainted with the bacteria she lived with. Move the mother to a new environment, such as a hospital, and there was actually more risk involved. As hospital sterilization procedures changed, that became less of a factor.

The disadvantages to home births were very sobering. "Holding a newborn's hand growing cold with the dew of death is a very difficult thing; you may be glad that you're there to help, but it's not fun," he remarked.

Siebenmorgen delivered all three of his own children and many of his grandchildren. He joked that it was his way of getting into the birthing room.

61

Treating the Eternal

Siebenmorgen was regularly called upon to deliver speeches to first-year medical students. More often than not, he reminded them that treating the ill was not always about the medicine and the technology.

"Treat that which is eternal in all of us," he told them. "That's what medicine is all about. It's not always just about the drugs and the X-rays and the numbers. It's about people. It's not something taught regularly in the medical schools."

One example recounted for the students' benefit told of an elderly woman who called on Siebenmorgen to make a house call. She was living in the old Deming Hotel, a grand structure that had been transformed into apartments for the elderly. When he arrived, the room was dark and dingy. The woman was very ill and she knew it. When he was done treating her medically, she asked that he treat her soul.

"She said, 'I know you go to church. Would you mind sitting down here with me and repeating the First Psalm with me?'"

"By God, I'm glad I knew it," he recalled.

So he recited it with her: "Blessed is the man that walketh not in the counsel of the ungodly, nor standeth in the way of sinners."

By the end of the recitation she was smiling.

After fifty-three years of practice, Siebenmorgen knew what was important. He knew that while his medical skill and training would help him achieve his mission, deep down the real mission was treating the eternal.

62

A Memorable Surgery

William Ritchie, MD, was born on September 14, 1923, and spent his childhood in Evansville, Indiana, and Palm Beach, Florida. He received his bachelor of science in anatomy and physiology from Indiana University in 1945. He then continued his studies at the IU School of Medicine, graduating in 1948. Ritchie completed a rotating internship at Ball Memorial Hospital in Muncie, Indiana, before entering practice in July 1949.

After practicing in a partnership for two years, Ritchie began working as a solo physician in 1951. His practice included general medicine, major and minor surgery, and obstetrics. He also served in the U.S. Air Force, working as a flight surgeon, and although he retired in 2004, he still practices aviation medicine.

Ritchie has held many positions within the Indiana Academy of Family Physicians, including president from 1979 to 1980.

As mentioned in other stories, it was not uncommon for family physicians, especially in rural areas, to perform major surgery. Many did tonsillectomies and appendectomies, but others did more extensive procedures. Ritchie was one of those doctors who received such training and made surgery part of his practice.

During my internship I contacted a doctor here in Evansville that I knew because I caddied for him and had occasionally played golf with him. I had wanted a surgical residency. The war had ended, and all the guys coming back from the service had preference. You couldn't buy a surgical residency at that time. I wrote letter after letter and never heard back from any of them.

Finally, a doctor from Milwaukee wrote to me and told me that on the day he had received my letter, he received enough applications to fill their quota for the next ten years. So a friend of mine suggested that I talk to this doctor I knew and ask about working with him and learning surgery, so I did. I asked if I could be a paid assistant. He said, "Let me tell you what I want and see what you think. You would be like a junior partner." That sounded better than a paid assistant, so I went into partnership with him, and my salary was progressively increased to the point that we were equal in three or five years. I assisted in all the surgeries, and if I had the case, I did it, and he would assist and teach me. Then, I got called into the service, and when I came back I went solo. I did my own belly surgeries including gallbladders and appendectomies, tonsils, hemorrhoids, and GYN surgeries. I didn't do much

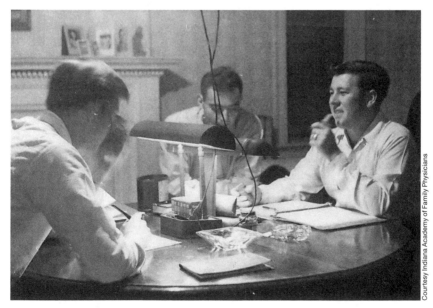

William Ritchie (right)

intestinal work. I did thyroidectomies and hernias. I didn't do any operative orthopedics, but I did closed orthopedic procedures. And I did obstetrics.

When it got to the point that I could not make enough money doing obstetrical work to pay the insurance premiums, even though I dearly loved it, I had to quit. Then they started putting limitations on the surgeries we could do, and again insurance premiums were on the rise. And so many surgeons were arriving on the scene; I decided it wasn't financially worth it anymore. So I quit that too.

Family docs don't do much surgery anymore. We sure had a lot of fun practicing medicine back then.

Ritchie recalls one of his most memorable, if not most unusual, surgical "emergencies":

I had an old guy whose wife called one night after my wife and I had just returned home from a movie. She wanted to know if I made house calls, and I said I could, if necessary.

She said, "My husband's bleeding, and I can't get it stopped."

Immediately, I was thinking nosebleed, and said, "From where is he bleeding."

She hemmed and hawed and said, "He's bleeding from his genitals."

I told her I couldn't take care of that in the home and she should take him to the ER, and I could meet them there. This guy had tried to circumcise himself with a pair of scissors and a razorblade at 3:00 in the afternoon. This is now 10:30 at night.

It took me longer to unwrap this package than it did to complete the job. The first thing he did, of all things, was to wrap cotton around it, and then a couple of washcloths, and then two bath towels around it too. He was bleeding through the bath towels. I kept him in the hospital overnight because I didn't know how much blood he had lost.

He was a great big guy, about sixty-three years old. I went out to the waiting room to talk to his wife and said, "Your husband, does he drink?"

She said, "He's never had a drink in his life."

"Why did he do it?"

"He's a hard-headed Dutchman who thinks he can do anything and you can't tell him any different. He's bashful, and he didn't want to go to the doctor to have this done so he decided to do it himself."

By this time, he's lying on a table in the ER with a parade of staff going through there once the word got out. The only thing I could do was to complete the job. So, I'm sewing it up and talking to him. I said, "You know once we finish this, you can't use this for a couple of weeks until this heals up really well."

"Well doctor, I'll try, but I wake up every morning with the biggest erection you ever saw."

I said, "Nurse, could I have some more sutures please?" And I put another extra row of stitches in between the ones that I had done already.

63

The Indiana University School of Medicine
The Days of the Medical School Pyramid

Alvin Haley, MD, was born on November 2, 1926, and grew up in Fort Wayne, Indiana. Before college, he was in the U.S. Navy Reserves, serving on active duty from 1945 to 1946. He attended Indiana University, graduating in 1950 with a bachelor of science in anatomy and physiology. He also attended IU for medical school, graduating in 1953. Haley finished an internship at Lutheran Hospital in Fort Wayne in 1954 before entering a practice that included obstetrics. He has worked in both partnerships and group practices.

Haley is an emeritus professor of family medicine at the IU School of Medicine and former director of the family medicine residency program at Methodist Hospital in Indianapolis. He served as president of the Indiana Academy of Family Physicians from 1969 to 1970. He retired from family medicine in August 1997.

It is unquestionably very difficult to get into medical school today. It's extremely competitive and only the very top students qualify. But once in, medical schools make every effort to assist students in successfully getting through the extensive and difficult course of studies. It's different today than it was in the mid-twentieth century.

The author remembers that his father, Max Feldman, MD, who attended medical school in Switzerland in the mid-1930s, told him that he did not see a single test until the end of two years of study. The big test came and if you failed it, that was the end of your medical school training. They kicked you out. Your medical career was over.

Hoosier family doctors who attended medical school during the 1940s and 1950s recall the harsh inhospitable atmosphere of the IU School of Medicine. During interviews for this book Ritchie, Haley, and several other physicians recounted that on the first day of medical school, the medical school's dean would come down to Bloomington from Indianapolis to address the incoming class. Haley remembers:

There were 150 in our class, and my recollection is that Dean John Van Nuys told us that it was the intention of the medical school to graduate all 150 of us. But we all knew better. In prior years, the deans admonished the new medical students to look to the person on their left and then on their right, and then would say, "One of you three are not going to make it to Indianapolis." In other words, the first year was to screen out those that were not as talented.

I started medical school in 1949 in Bloomington. At the time, I had a girlfriend who lived in one of the houses along Third Street. Also living in that house was a girl named Jean who was a classmate of mine in high school. I was walking with them one day, and Jean turned to my girlfriend and said, "Do you understand that you are

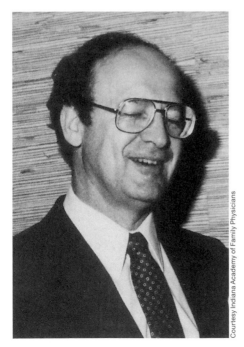

Courtesy Indiana Academy of Family Physicians

Alvin Haley

jeopardizing Al's career by taking up his time." That's indicative of the amount of attention that we thought we had to give to medical school classes and studying to survive.

Ritchie, who attended medical school a number of years before Haley, also remembers medical school as a similar situation:

My father impressed on me that becoming a doctor was the thing I should try to do. I thought he was right, and I really didn't consider anything else. I did my premed at Indiana University, Bloomington, and then med school at IU as well.

Freshman year of med school was considered "flunk out" year at that time. I don't think it's that way any longer because of the need for more physicians. They really weeded out the chaff. They intended to do it, and we knew it. You were really under the gun.

I started at Bloomington in 1941 and was exempt from the draft on an education deferment until I got into medical school, and then they drafted many of us. We really had to put out, or we were going to be marching, digging trenches, or sailing the high seas, or who knows what. One-third of our class was army, one-third navy, and one-third civilians.

We left Bloomington for Indianapolis for the sophomore year. The pressure was still on, but we knew that the flunk-out rate was greatly reduced. Completing the sophomore year, you let out a great big sigh of relief that you were going to become a physician. They began to treat you like one at that point. And, of course, during the senior year we were referred to as doctor.

Nowadays, I think that the problem of getting into the field of medicine occurs long before medical school. You have to get top grades and do well on the entrance exam. Once you make it in medical school, just do good work and forget about it. In four years you are going to be given an MD degree. The question nowadays is, "can I get into medical school." Back then, you did have to fight like hell to get in, but then you also had to fight like hell to stay in school for a couple of years. We started with 110 at Bloomington, which was down a bit because of the war, and we sent ninety-seven or ninety-eight to Indianapolis. We picked up a few that had been dropped from previous classes in their second year, and then they were admitted back to repeat that year and went on with us.

My class had folks from everywhere because it was wartime, and they were shipped there by the military. We had people from all over the United States. But generally in the years surrounding the war, it was a little difficult to get into medical school at IU if you didn't go to IU for undergrad. You really had to be a hotshot to get accepted because they gave preference to their own students. If you went to Wabash or DePauw, it carried a little weight because of the scholastic records of those schools, but you still had to be really good. And you had to be a damn genius to get into IU from out of state.

Actually, I was accepted to medical school twice. I was accepted for the class ahead of me, and I contracted acute glomerulonephritis and had to drop out. I took incompletes, and knew that I would have to go back and finish up. Of course, I didn't know what I was supposed to do, so I reapplied. Then they put me through the same procedure with interviews.

I went into my interview, and this austere looking guy was sitting there with my folder in his hands. He opened it up and said, "It says here you were accepted for last year's class. Why didn't you go?" So I told him what had occurred and he said, "This is a waste of my time. If you are accepted once you are accepted. Get out of here." I came about three feet off the ground.

64

An Expensive House Call

Fred Blix, MD, was born on January 8, 1918, and grew up in north-west Chicago. He attended the University of Illinois, Urbana, receiving his bachelor of arts in chemistry in 1940. He attended the University of Illinois, Chicago, for his doctor of medicine degree, graduating in 1943. In 1942 he enlisted in the U.S. Army's Specialized Training Program, but deactivated his service until after his internship at Lutheran Deaconess Hospital, now Lutheran General Hospital, in Chicago. After serving with the army and a deployment overseas, Blix returned to Ladoga, Indiana, where he started private practice, including obstetrics, before relocating to Crawfordsville, Indiana, where he continued his family practice career.

He retired from private practice in 1974 but then began working for Saint Vincent Hospital in Indianapolis as the director of the Family Medicine Residency until 1982. He then served as the director of the Chemical Dependency Unit of the Saint Vincent Stress Center until 1988. He began doing locum tenens in Indiana, Kentucky, and Arizona before retiring from the practice of medicine in 1996. Blix also received a faculty appointment in the Department of Family Medicine at the Indiana University School of Medicine as a volunteer clinical associate professor. He served as president of the Indiana Academy of Family Physicians from 1975 to 1976. Blix lives in Zionsville with his wife, Marjorie.

Blix once won a girl's heart with a nickel. He remembers dating the girl who would become his wife while he was in the process of completing his nine-month internship. On one of their six dates before he proposed, Blix passed a machine offering bags of salted peanuts for five cents. He dug deep into his pocket, retrieved a nickel, and bought a bag of peanuts for them to share. For medical students in the 1940s this was quite an extravagance. "I was impressed," recalls his wife, Marge. "I thought, 'Boy! He has money to throw around!'"

After marrying Marge and opening his own practice in Ladoga, Indiana, Blix was able to afford a little more than just the occasional bag of peanuts—a house to live in, for example, and an office to rent for his practice. Equipment and an examining table followed shortly after.

Just because he owned his own practice did not mean he was financially home free. He recalls a story about a particular house call that taught him a thing or two about the financial aspects of family medicine at that time:

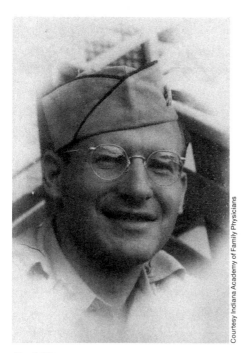

Courtesy Indiana Academy of Family Physicians

Fred Blix

I learned some economics lessons in the process of starting my career. I'll never forget one rainy night when I was called out for a house call way out in the middle of the country. I got in my old car and, you know, the roads out to the house were pretty good really. They were paved, which was kind of something special back then. Not many of the roads around Ladoga were paved when I started practicing. It could sometimes be really difficult trying to get to a house call.

So, I got to the house and I thought well, I'd better just park off the road a little ways. Better to be safe and leave some room on the road. So that's what I did. I pulled my car into the grass a little ways and went on into the house.

Big mistake. I could feel the tires sinking down into the ground even as I put the car in park. And shoot, there just wasn't anything I could do about that. I needed to get inside and see the patient. So, I just left the car and went in and saw the patient. I fixed him up, charged him eight dollars for the visit, and was on my way.

Afterward, I called a wrecker to come pull me out of the mud. And you know what? The darned thing cost me fifteen dollars!

65

Welcome to Town, Doc

When Blix opened his medical practice in 1947 it was a much different time. He was the only family doctor in the community of a thousand people. As he drove his car and trailer into town from Chicago he was not expecting to inherit a family, but that is exactly what he got. He remembers fondly the experience of starting a practice in small-town Indiana:

My wife, Marge, and I loaded all our possessions into a little trailer, hooked it up to the car, and headed out of Chicago down to Ladoga, Indiana. I thought we had a lot of stuff, so I rented a four-wheeler trailer—you know, the kind where the front wheels would turn.

I remember coming down the hill into Crawfordsville. The four-wheeler trailer? That was a bad idea. It started swaying back and forth, and boy, I put the brakes on very gingerly. Anyway, we sailed into Ladoga all right. And there we were, two newlyweds rattling around in a big old house. It was way too big. We were renting from a surgeon in Crawfordsville who heard we were coming. We didn't know a soul in town.

But the two of us got settled there as best we could, and I went on into work on my first day. I'll always remember my first patient on my very first day was the town banker. I tried talking to him to find out what was wrong with him, but eventually I realized all he was doing was trying to be sure I had somebody to see that day. That was the first day of October 1947.

Well, I had two other patients come in that day and I'm pretty sure they were there for somewhat the same reason. I think they were conscious of getting me going and getting started. They sure wanted a doctor badly down in Ladoga.

Marge remembers being welcomed by the community as well as her husband, even though she stayed home to raise the family:

The whole community just picked us up, and really you couldn't have asked for anything better. They were just plain friendly. People were always stopping by, and when our oldest son was born in February of that year, they brought us gifts and food.

I remember one of the women invited me to a group of women that she was having over for an afternoon meeting. Her home was within walking distance of us, so I walked over and they were very gracious and so nice to me. One woman asked me if I had a sewing machine and I said, "Well, no I don't," and she said, "Well, anytime you want to sew something you come on over." They were just, just nice.

Occasionally Fred's patients would call the house when I was there. "I don't want to bother doc at the office," they'd say. And they would want a prescription or something. Of course, I'd tell them I couldn't do anything, but I would listen and Fred would write up a prescription right there. He didn't charge them. He just wrote the prescription and they picked it up. It was a good thing for a lot of people.

We really got to know the people in town, and we got to love them. We both did. For six years we had the office on the first floor of our house, and we had an apartment where we lived on the top. Patients would frequently come to our front door. It was just that they felt comfortable with us. They knew us.

Nowadays we live out of town, but whenever there's a funeral or a birthday party down there for someone, we always go down to Ladoga. So many times we've walked through the door and people have said, "Oh! Here's Doc and Marge. Here's Doc and Marge." Fred will always be the doc. Their doc. That'll never change.

66

Maria

Occasionally, in the life and career of a family physician, a special patient comes along and touches that doctor's life. There are always a few patients over the span of a lifelong career that the doctor is unable to forget. For Blix, one of those patients is named Maria. He remembers the first time she came into his office, and how he has stayed connected to her throughout the rest of her life:

This particular patient, Maria, was living with her stepfather when I first met her. She came into the office and she really was a tremulous girl—afraid of people, just afraid of people. She'd been told often that she wasn't worth anything and she had been told, "You can never do anything." She came to me because, well, she obviously wasn't feeling too good. I had her sit down, and I listened to her heart, and asked her what the problem was and how was she feeling. She just poured it out. She told me about her stepfather and her situation and how bad she felt about herself. She told me she felt like she couldn't do anything, and she felt like she wasn't worth anything.

What did I do? I sat and listened to her. I let her speak for as long as she needed and I never interrupted her. Once she'd gotten everything off of her chest, I just looked her in the eyes and said simply, "Maria, you're perfectly healthy. You can do anything you want to do." That's it. She paused for a moment, and then I saw that an idea had come into her head. She looked pretty timid, and she asked me very quietly, "Doc?"

"Yes," I said.

"Do you suppose I could get a job here at the hospital?"

"Well, I don't see why not."

And that's what she did. First, they let her pass the water around, and then she got to work in the nursery. And when she got that job in the nursery, boy, she was in seventh heaven. She just loved those little babies. She loved them to pieces.

She worked there at the hospital for a long time. After a while, I could see her demeanor start to change. She walked up straighter and she spoke clearer. Gradually she started to feel better about herself. She started to feel like she was worth something. A few years later, she met a very nice young man and got married, and they're still very happy together. Over the years every time my wife and I have seen her she's been so excited about life and so happy to see us.

Well, I really do feel like I helped her. And you know what she tells me? To this day—she tells me she thinks I'm God! I'm not God. I'm just a family doc who took the time and cared enough to listen.

67

Some of the Best Lessons Are the Ones You Teach Yourself

As a general practitioner, Blix remembers teaching himself many elements of the practice of medicine and patient care. Although he attended medical school and completed a nine-month internship (the standard duration for an internship at that time), as he puts it, "It wasn't a very comprehensive education where you sit in class and discuss things like they do now." And the extensive clinical training that occurs today prior to starting practice was generally lacking then for those going into general primary care medicine.

Blix remembers his internship involving simple tasks such as bringing patients to the operating table on a gurney. His time in the military as a medical officer was not very helpful either. He recalls, "You didn't see patients a lot because they were all healthy buzzards."

After the war ended, Blix began his own small-town practice. Because of the nature and duration of his training, not to mention the time he spent away from school during the war, Blix sometimes had to do a bit of improvisation when it came to medical procedures and techniques. He remembers frequently excusing himself from a visit with a patient to sneak off into the hallway and look something up in one of his medical textbooks.

However, the most important lesson Blix learned could not be found in any of his textbooks—listening. He recalls the significant effect his listening had on his patients:

When I was practicing, that's just the way things were in medicine. You got to know these people and you were sympathetic. You didn't have to cure a lot of the people, really. A lot of their problems eventually went away on their own. But simply listening—that's what worked wonders. With older people, particularly women, I found that if you just listened to what they complained about, they were so thankful. And it made all the difference in the world.

It seemed like a good thing to do for a patient before surgery, too. It put them at ease. Every time I was responsible for a patient entering surgery, I would enter their name into my little notebook, and I would diligently go back and see them the next day, and the next day, and the next day, and so on. Just say, you know, "How's it going?"

"Fine," they'd say. That's all it took. But it meant so much to my patients. And I believe it really helped them get better when they were sick.

I remember a particular experience in Yuma, Arizona, when my wife, Marge, and I were out there on a trip. We were staying in an RV park, and I noticed a woman sitting out front of her RV, just two down from us. She was waiting while her husband was in surgery. I didn't know her from Adam, but I just sat down with her for a spell. That's all I did. I think we maybe shared some coffee until he got out, but we didn't talk a whole lot. Just sat. I just kept her company.

And you know, she still sends us long letters about what's going on in that RV park every Christmas. It's been so many years now. I don't think she ever forgot that.

Sometimes all you can do is just sit with a patient. Sit or listen. Or cry together. When they lose somebody, you cry. I never once failed to at least pull out my stethoscope and listen to the heart. Take the pulse. Just a simple touch is a miraculously healing thing.

Yes, I had to teach myself many things in practice that I just didn't have the opportunity to learn in medical school or internship. That's just the way it was back then. You learned from experience. For instance, my office was on the second floor. I developed a theory that if a patient made it up there his cardiovascular system couldn't be too bad! Of course, I never told them that, but it seemed to hold true!

But listening, listening was the most important lesson I taught myself, by far.

68

The Right Answer

Eugene Gillum, MD, was born on August 12, 1920, and grew up in Randolph County, Indiana. He received his bachelor of science from Tri-State College in Angola, Indiana, in 1942 and another bachelor of science degree from Earlham College in Richmond, Indiana, in 1949. He attended the Indiana University School of Medicine, graduating in 1953. He served in the U.S. Army Air Corps during World War II.

Gillum entered family medicine in 1954 and worked in Portland, Indiana, in solo practice. His career included the full range of family medicine, obstetrics, and assisting with surgery. He received a faculty appointment in the Department of Family Medicine at the IU School of Medicine as a volunteer clinical instructor and has served as a Jay County health officer for thirty-six years. He was the chairman of the Indiana Association of Public Health Physicians for thirteen years. He retired from practice in 1992.

Gillum faced some unusual situations in his medical career but possibly none more threatening than the following episode. And he lived to tell the tale!

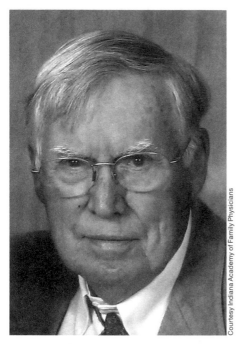

Courtesy Indiana Academy of Family Physicians

Eugene Gillum

Well, I had one lady that lived out in the country, five or six miles. She had a belly-ache and I went out to see her on a house call one night. After examining her, I decided that she had appendicitis. I brought her in to the hospital and notified the surgeon and anesthesiologist. We took her appendix out without any problems.

I walked down to the waiting room after we were all done with the surgery to talk to the husband who was a big, tall guy with bib overalls and floppy hat.

I said, "Well, we got her done. We took her appendix out and she's going to be all right."

He said, "Well, I'm glad."

At that moment, I noticed that he was putting the .32-caliber pistol that he had in his hand into his pocket. We had some crazy guys like that. I was glad I brought the right message to him—the one he wanted to hear.

69

The Back-Door Approach

Gillium understood there were times when things were done differently in the country. Knowing that, here is how he finessed house calls to create the best results for his patients:

Years ago, we were flying out to see my sister in California, and a guy sitting next to me on the plane said, "What kind of a doctor are you?" I said, "I'm a back-door specialist." He asked me what I meant. Let me tell you why I told him that:

At that time, making house calls was still a popular thing to do. We didn't have an ambulance service, and if you were too sick to go the hospital, then the doctor had to go see you.

I got a call at 10:00 at night, and there was a man that was eighty-two years old with a temperature of 102 and coughing and feeling terrible. He lived four miles out in the country. I had never seen him before, but I had to go see him to see what he needed. Well, you can just about guess that this old boy had pneumonia, and that he was in trouble.

When you're in the country, and you go out to make a house call, you don't ever enter through the front door. If you are accepted by the community, you always go in and out of the back door. It was also an important thing to do from a medical standpoint. When you entered the back door, you'd see how many cats and dogs were hanging out in the yard, and how many cases of beer or Coke were on the back porch. You'd then go through the kitchen to see what's on the kitchen table, see what kind of medicine and stuff was sitting on the window sill; go past the bathroom and see what's sitting on the back of the toilet, and see the general organization in the home. By the time you got to the bedroom to see the patient, you knew a lot of information about the living situation.

So, in this case I said to this man, "You have pneumonia and I need you in the hospital."

Sure enough as I expected, he said, "Doc, I ain't going to that damned death house." That was the term that they commonly used back then. Even so, I knew I had to get him to the hospital, but he wasn't going to go.

So, I replied, "Mr. Jones, I think you need to go to the hospital. Let's do it this way. I'm going to start you on some medicine and by 10:00 tomorrow morning, if you aren't feeling better, somebody in the family should call me. If you are better, fine. If not, or if I have any doubts about your condition, I'll have to put you in the hospital and get an X-ray." The patient agreed to the deal.

That judgment was based on what I had seen around the house before I ever saw the patient. From what I observed in the house, there wasn't anyone there who could intelligently or reliably report to me if he's got a temperature, and really tell me on the phone if he is better or worse. Nothing I saw in the house made me think this was a good situation, and that he could be properly cared for there. I stole twelve hours but still put him in the hospital the next day where he belonged.

So, if you made a house call in the big city, and you went in and out the back door, what would happen? Somebody would shoot you! You wouldn't go in and out of the back door in Indianapolis. But in the country, that's the way it was done. It was comfortable doing it that way.

70

The Ten-Dollar Delivery

Phyllis Grant, MD, was born on October 31, 1925. She attended Indiana University, where she received her bachelor of arts degree in 1945 and her medical degree in 1953. Grant completed an internship at the Indianapolis City Hospital. She entered practice in 1954, working in New Castle, Indiana.

Although she initially practiced in a partnership, Grant spent most of her career working as a solo physician beginning in 1965. Her practice included obstetrics and assisting in surgery. A highlight from her career is that she has delivered 2,365 babies. Grant retired in 2003.

In the 1950s, doctors did not have to charge as much money for a checkup or a service as they do now. It was typical for a visit to the doctor's office to cost about two dollars, while a house call cost three dollars. And while doctors were still interns and worked for a hospital to gain the valuable educational experience, of course, they did not charge patients for their services.

So, as an intern, Grant was not allowed to accept payment from patients. Regardless, she enjoyed treating patients with all sorts of maladies, but she especially loved delivering babies. Despite the regulations surrounding her internship, there was one patient, she remembers, who was determined to give her something for her services:

When I was still interning in 1953, one of the first home-delivery house calls that I ever made was in Indianapolis, near the general area of where Wishard Hospital is now. Most babies were delivered in the hospital back in those days; Wishard was really busy with obstetrics back then. But this young woman was having some trouble with her delivery, so I went out to do a home delivery. We rode the ambulance over from the hospital. When I got there, she was upstairs in bed, and her father was by her side.

I spent a total of about two hours at her home helping this young woman with her delivery. Her father was there, constantly near her, helping take care of her and wanting to make sure everything was okay.

During the delivery there were also a whole bunch of little kids that kept peeking around the door to where the young woman was, trying to see what was going on. One head on top of the other. There were about four or five of them, and they weren't her children. I don't know if they were siblings or nieces or nephews or what. But the father of the young woman in labor kept shooing them back out so that we could continue.

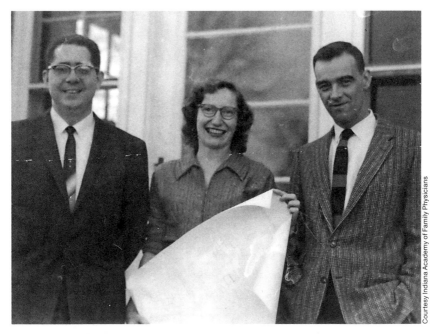

Phyllis Grant (center)

Courtesy Indiana Academy of Family Physicians

But they would come back, and he would shoo them out again, and we would get on with the delivery.

So, I was there for about two hours, and eventually we got this young woman's baby delivered. I got her some fluids and took care of everything that needed to be done. I then packed up and was ready to leave. I told her she just needed to rest and enjoy spending some time with her new baby.

But before I could leave the father took a ten-dollar bill out of his billfold and just insisted on giving it to me. I told him, "Well, I can't take that." I was an intern; I wasn't allowed to accept payment. But he told me, "You just have to take this money. You just don't know how much we appreciate it." I didn't know what else to do, so I took it, even though I wasn't supposed to.

So that was my first delivery—for ten dollars. But you know, I really enjoyed delivering that baby, and I was happy to do it for free.

71

I Recognize Your Face
But I Sure Don't Know Your Name

Grant enjoyed getting to know her patients. Today, nurse practitioners or physician assistants may take care of many patients' visits and physicians are pressed to see many patients quickly. But Grant was fortunate to practice at a time when physicians were able to spend the time necessary to know her patients really well, and she liked that.

"It was fun," she says of the old days. "I mean, you got to know patients back then and you had time to listen and talk to them, and learn about their families and their problems." She continues, "Later there was more paperwork and more rules and regulations. I don't think any doctor has time to just sit down and listen and just talk with people anymore. There are rules and regulations and malpractice that you have to worry about."

She remembers, with a mixture of fondness and lighthearted irritation, the experience of being constantly approached by patients asking for a quick diagnosis at the grocery store or a restaurant:

I got recognized all over town. I still do, as a matter of fact. Though now people just want to say hello, when I was practicing they always had a question of one sort or another about their health. When I was still practicing, I just didn't eat at restaurants in town because I just couldn't get through a meal. As soon as I sat down, somebody would come up and say their ear hurt, or ask what they could do about this pain in their leg, or ask how they should treat one thing or another. I'd try to be halfway decent and tell them to take two aspirin and go to bed; or call me the next day and make an appointment. And sometimes, I would say, "put ice on it" or something like that, but the questions were just constant. It got to be overwhelming for me, so I started eating out in Muncie or Anderson, or Indianapolis. And I did lots of grocery shopping at midnight!

As my pediatric patients got older and I saw more patients, more and more people began coming up to me. I would really get recognized all over town. They were either people I treated a few times, or people I treated as children who had since grown up. I couldn't keep track of all of them, especially the ones I treated as children or delivered. And, of course, it was great fun to watch how they grew. But then big adults might come up to me at a restaurant in town and say, "How are you?" or "You used to give me those shots when I was a kid that hurt so bad!"

I always responded, "Well, I recognize your face, but I sure don't know your name." That was my stock response; still is. Though, now that I'm not practicing anymore people just say "Hello." So now I can go out to eat in New Castle.

I remember one woman I saw who had an ulcerative colitis, which can be made much worse with stress. I tried to treat her and eventually referred her to a specialist. She moved away for nine years, and when she came back, I ran into her in the grocery store in town. She introduced herself and said, "When you treated me, I had ulcerative colitis that was so bad. You were so good to me, Doctor Grant." We got to catching up, and she told me that just before her colitis went away, she'd gotten a divorce. I said to her, "Well, I think you divorced your colitis!"

72

I'm a Doctor, I Promise

When Grant entered medical school and started practicing medicine in the mid-1950s, it was uncommon for a woman to be a doctor. Most women in the medical field were nurses, though Grant never considered another career path. Her mother's cousin was a general practitioner long before Grant started studying to become one herself. That influenced her to believe that there was nothing strange in becoming a "lady doctor," as they were often called back then.

Grant remembers her second grade teacher going around the class-room asking each student what they wanted to be when they grew up. She said that she wanted to be a medical doctor, and she never considered anything else from that day on.

She recalls that there were ten girls in her medical school class at Indiana University out of about two hundred total students. "Nine of us graduated." She says that some of the other girls used to feel awkward or insecure around their male classmates, but Grant never did. "I just have a different personality, I guess." She said if her male classmates caught a female blushing they would tease the girl about it and make her feel

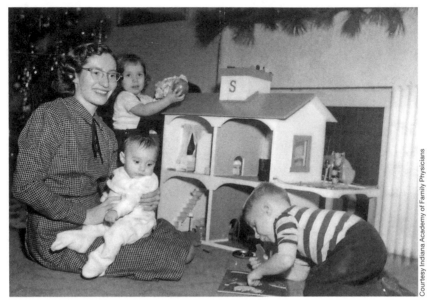

Courtesy Indiana Academy of Family Physicians

Grant with her children at Christmas.

uncomfortable. "But they never did bother me," Grant remembers.

Often mistaken for a nurse at hospitals, she never let the confusion bother her or bring her down. "I never felt imposed on or mistreated. If somebody felt I wasn't as good as they were, or shouldn't be a doctor because I was a woman, then I just let it brush off my back. I didn't pay any attention," she said. While Grant hardly ever felt challenged or mistreated by fellow male doctors, she does remember one uncomfortable encounter with a female nurse:

"I'm positive I was the only female doctor in Henry County. I was working in New Castle in a practice I had with two of my male doctor friends. We had privileges at the state hospital in Indianapolis so we could admit our sick patients there if they needed to be hospitalized.

"I remember at one point in the 1960s I was taking care of a young patient who I had brought to the pediatric unit of the hospital. As I went in to check on her one day with her patient chart in my hand, I heard a harsh, hoity voice behind me demand curtly, 'What are you doing with her chart?'

"A nurse had come up behind me and was standing over me with her hands on her hips. She was demanding to know what I was doing with my patient's chart. She must have thought I was the girl's mother or something.

"I just simply said I was the patient's doctor, and that took care of that. "Every now and then I see that nurse, at the grocery or something, and she says to me, 'I just remember how rude I was to you that day at the hospital! I had no idea you were a doctor.'

"I tell her it's all right. No reason to get upset. It didn't bother me then, and it doesn't bother me now; I just corrected her and went on with doing my job. The job of being a family doctor is the same privilege for a woman as it is for a man."

73

Famished

Frank Beardsley Jr., MD, was born on July 8, 1925, and was raised in Frankfort, Indiana. He served in the U.S. Navy from July 1943 to July 1946, and deployed overseas in January 1946. He received his undergraduate degree from Wabash College in 1949 and then attended the Indiana University School of Medicine, graduating in 1954. He served an internship at Indianapolis City Hospital from July 1954 to July 1955.

Beardsley was in a solo practice from 1955 until 1972, when Frankfort Medical Clinic opened, continuing his practice with four other physicians. He practiced pediatrics, adult medicine, and geriatrics and delivered about two thousand babies. Beardsley administered anesthesia, performed minor surgery, and did limited orthopedics until his retirement in 1991. He lives in Frankfort with his wife, Maryann.

Beardsley recalls an endearing patient who had some difficulty understanding the medical jargon spoken during a medical procedure:

I once had this patient named Silvia who was mildly mentally handicapped and had a speech impediment. She was a sweet person and we all really liked her.

She was having some problems with her stomach, and so I ordered an upper GI. Doctor Williams was the radiologist at that time. She was a heavy woman and loved to eat, but had to be NPO (nothing by mouth) until the procedure. This was the busiest day in fluoroscopy that Doctor Williams ever had, so he didn't get to poor Silvia until late in the afternoon. She was one hungry patient. But we couldn't give her anything until after the procedure was completed.

Now, the heavier the patient, the more milligrams of sedative they need. So, here was Silvia starving to death and here is Doctor Williams looking through the fluoroscope in the darkened room. She needed more medication.

He says to the tech, "Give me three mils," and Silvia said, "bweakfast, wunch, and tupper."

74

Memorable Victories

Kenneth Gray, MD, was born on February 14, 1934, and grew up in Indiana, Illinois, and Wisconsin. He received his bachelor of arts degree from Butler University in Indianapolis, Indiana, in 1956. He received his doctor of medicine degree from the Indiana University School of Medicine in 1959. He completed a rotating internship and one year of internal medicine residency at Methodist Hospital in Indianapolis. Additionally, Gray served in the Indiana National Guard.

Gray entered practice in 1961, working as a solo practitioner. He delivered babies and was the team physician for Speedway High School. He also served as medical director at Robin Run Village Healthcare. Gray retired from family medicine in 1999.

As with most of the family doctors interviewed, Gray recounts some memorable house calls. It is a great source of stories from the physicians of that era. When doctors entered a patient's home, they could be faced with almost anything, from routine ailments to acute heart attacks. It is hard to imagine today with ambulance services readily available and fully staffed emergency departments, but they would see true emergencies right there in the home.

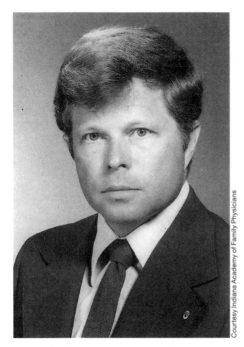

Courtesy Indiana Academy of Family Physicians

Kenneth Gray

I made a lot of house calls in my career. It was just part of a family doctor's practice routine back then. I saw all kinds of things. I remember once that I was doing a pelvic exam in the office. Her legs were spread apart, and I was just ready to insert the speculum. My nurse came to the door and said, "A patient's wife is on the phone, and she thinks she has an emergency."

It was another patient who lived about two blocks from the office, and her husband was having tremendous abdominal pain, which came on suddenly. This sounded bad to me, so I literally left this woman in the stirrups, and I went to see him. He had a critical acute abdomen, and I made the diagnosis of a ruptured abdominal aortic aneurysm. I sent him to the emergency room and got him admitted immediately.

At Methodist Hospital at that time, surgery rooms were sort of open, as you could walk by the door in the hall and talk to the surgeons. So, I went up to surgery and told the vascular surgeon that I needed him as soon as he could possibly get away. He came down, and I could tell from his attitude that he was irritated that this young upstart family doctor would come up to surgery and demand his service. The patient went to surgery and he lived. To have somebody with a ruptured aortic aneurysm at home and go through that and live was practically unheard of.

Coincidentally, the lady that I left in stirrups and the patient with the aneurysm were close friends. Their families were traveling partners. I guess in retrospect, she didn't mind being left in the stirrups. A happy outcome for everyone.

One of the most memorable house calls I ever made was in Haughville in Indianapolis just west of the medical center. I was told the patient was near death. I was ushered into the room. The elderly lady was lying in bed and nonresponsive. There was a candle lit by the side of the bed. What a grim scene.

The priest was there to administer last rites. I got a history from the family that she was diabetic and had slept through her lunch. I had seen lots of people with hypoglycemia; the summer before I started medical school, I worked in a sanitarium where I assisted in performing insulin shock therapy on depressed patients. Examining her clinical appearance, she had a familiar look to me. I pulled out an ampule of 50 percent dextrose, which I gave her intravenously. In a moment, she fluttered her eyelids and sat up in bed like Lazarus. She was alive, alert, and just fine! You can imagine how everyone looked at her in amazement.

I made a house call one time and got paid with a bag of Roma tomatoes. What a wonderful time to practice medicine!

75

A Late-Night Phone Call

In the days before minute clinics, urgent care centers, and fully staffed emergency rooms, it was not uncommon for family doctors to meet patients at their office or nearby emergency room when needed after hours. The son of a minister, Gray learned from a young age the value of going the extra mile for the sake of others.

In 1959, when Gray graduated from the Indiana University School of Medicine, he pursued what was then known as a general practice internship at Methodist Hospital in Indianapolis. Upon completion of this one-year internship, he could have elected to go into practice. But after rotating with a family doctor who was seeing more than fifty patients per day, Gray knew he needed more experience to serve his patients well. There was also a new general practice residency program at Methodist, intended to provide that additional experience. But "the fly in the ointment," said Gray, was that it essentially "existed only on paper." As such, he chose to do another year of internal medicine residency before entering private practice. It would only be a few short years before his willingness to further his medical education would serve Gray in a way he may not have foreseen.

"I've always felt treating patients over the telephone is a risk, a terrible risk," said Gray as he recalls a night like many others on call. "We don't realize how much we rely on the nuances of patient communication." These nuances cannot be taught in medical school. They can only be learned by observing patient after patient, as years of practice add up. "It's not so much what they say, but how they say it sometimes and the look on their faces," he explained.

"I remember one time, I had a lady call who was a good patient, a good mother," said Gray, his eyes fixed on some distant point as he recalls the details of an event that occurred more than three decades earlier. "She had a boy in junior high school. She said 'My boy's sick. His best friend is being treated for strep throat. Would you phone in a prescription for penicillin for him?'" Her voice was almost apologetic for having disturbed the doctor after what was certainly a long busy day at the office.

"My answer was 'no,'" he said, reciting a speech he had likely given hundreds or thousands of times over in his career, "I don't like to phone in prescriptions like that, but I'll sure be glad to check him." As part of the tight-knit community in Speedway, he knew the family well. "You know how close we live,' I told the mother. "I could meet you over at the office in five minutes." The office was a single-story brick building on High School Road where Gray saw patients for all but the first eighteen months of his career.

Her response was reassuring: "I really don't want to bother you." She spoke as though the five-minute trip would have been more trouble than it was worth for her respected physician.

"Well, that's fine," he replied, "but if he gets sicker and you want me to check him, you give me a call." He hung up the phone. Having known the family as his patients for some time, and having developed the relationship that comes with that kind of continuity of care, he was able to trust that the boy's mother would contact him as he instructed.

"Well, she called back in about fifteen minutes. 'He seems awfully sick, would you please check him?'" His voice echoed the concern that was present in hers. "Fine, I'll meet you at the office."

He beat the family to the office by a few minutes, and had the door unlocked and lights on when they arrived. "When the family arrived, the father was carrying this boy in. And this was a big kid," he recalled, "he weighed over a hundred pounds." The boy's sandy hair was pasted to his forehead by sweat, and as his father laid him gently on the exam table, his pajama top fell open.

"All the time, you worry, when something serious comes along will I recognize it?" said Gray, reflecting on the anxiety of uncertainty that often accompanies being a physician.

"Well, it took me about five seconds to make the diagnosis. This kid had meningococcemia." Meningococcemia is a potentially rapidly fatal infection of the blood that can kill within hours.

"So I just closed up his pajamas and said, 'Get back in the car, we're going to the emergency room.' Which we did." Upon arriving at the emergency room, he was treated appropriately with antibiotics and fully recovered.

"He played basketball in high school, so he had no residual effects from it," Gray said proudly. And then, as a tear formed in the corner of each of his light blue eyes, Gray relives the realization that struck him that night: "Had I called in his prescription for penicillin, I would have killed him." Instead, Gray had done the hard thing: He left his house, when he had rather have been sleeping, opened his office long after the hours posted on the door, and saved that boy's life.

76

If There Was Only an Instant Replay

Henry Webb Conrad, MD, was born on July 20, 1923, in Hamilton, Missouri. He attended Central Methodist College in Fayette, Missouri, receiving his bachelor's degree in chemistry. He then went on to the University of Louisville School of Medicine in 1944, receiving his medical degree in only two years.

While at the University of Louisville, he participated as a midshipman in a program designed to produce physicians quickly for World War II. He served in the U.S. Navy Reserves in World War II and in the U.S. Army Reserve Medical Corps during the Korean War.

Conrad began practicing medicine in 1948 after completing an internship at Louisville General Hospital in Kentucky. He worked both in a partnership and a solo practice during his forty-two years of family medicine in Milan and Lawrenceburg, Indiana. He served in many leadership hospital, medical professional, and community positions and was a charter fellow of the American Academy of Family Physicians. He retired in May 1990, relocating with his wife, Helen, to his hometown in Hamilton, Missouri, in 1993. They permanently moved to Florida in 2008, where Conrad died on July 10, 2010, after a full and distinguished career.

Conrad's practice included some surgical procedures and he delivered

1,713 babies. He was proud to say that he cared for multiple generations of families in this practice and that he "would not trade his life and career for anything."

Conrad saw plenty during a distinguished medical career. But he will probably be best remembered for what he did not see.

Conrad was a product of a unique U.S. Navy program that was designed to quickly produce commissioned medical officers for World War II. The V-12 program was rigorous. Participants had to maintain seventeen credit hours each semester and nine and a half hours of physical training each week. There were no summers off. Conrad earned his college and medical degrees in only five years. He served an internship at Louisville General Hospital before going into practice in Milan, Indiana. He later opened a clinic in Lawrenceburg, Indiana. Conrad, a charter fellow of the American Academy of Family Physicians, served the southeastern portion of Indiana and southwestern Ohio for forty-two years. He even delivered the first baby of 1960.

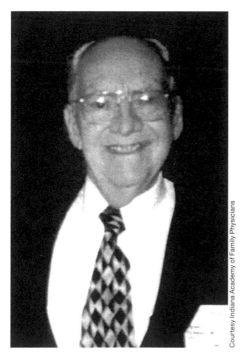

Conrad was also the team physician for one of the most famous basketball teams in high school history. The 1954 Milan Indians gained legendary status when they became the smallest high school to win the Indiana single-class state basketball championship. Enrollment that year was 161 students. The population of Milan: 1,200. The unlikely event was captured years later in the 1986 classic sports movie *Hoosiers.*

Courtesy Indiana Academy of Family Physicians

Henry Webb Conrad

The climax of the movie has the Milan team star character holding the basketball for a long time until there were only seconds to go on the game clock. In a slow-motion whirlwind, the star takes the final shot and seals the victory over the much larger, more athletic big-city school.

Conrad counted Milan team star Bobby Plump among the regular patients he treated from an early age. He followed the team through the sectional, regional, and semistate games, and the final showdown at the Butler Fieldhouse in Indianapolis.

Milan defeated Terre Haute Gerstmeyer in the afternoon of the Indiana State Basketball Championship Tournament. But the real drama occurred in the championship title game. The game was a defensive battle between Milan and the Muncie Central Bearcats. By the middle of the final quarter, the score was tied at only thirty points.

With more than four minutes left in the game, Plump decided to hold the ball, biding his time for a last-second shot. In this era before shot clocks and delay of game penalties, Plump stood there with the ball in hand. The crowd was slowly driven into a frenzy with each passing minute. Could this have been where the term "Hoosier Hysteria" originated?

The pressure was too much for a woman in the stands. Conrad rushed to the distressed woman's aid and while he was tending to her medical needs, Plump made his move and hit a fourteen-footer off the right side. The crowd roared. The scene was nothing less than pandemonium. In that moment, history was made.

Conrad missed seeing the title shot because he was attending to the woman.

Editor's Note: Conrad's wife, Helen, related this episode in the dedicated career of this family physician.

77

Grandma's Ailment

Gerald De Wester, MD, was born on December 12, 1929, and was raised in Roxana, Illinois. He attended Butler University for his undergraduate degree, graduating in 1955. De Wester then studied at the Indiana University School of Medicine, receiving his medical degree in 1959. He completed an internship at Methodist Hospital in Gary, Indiana, before establishing his practice in Indianapolis in 1960.

De Wester taught IU medical students and family medicine residents at Saint Francis Hospital in Beech Grove, Indiana (now known as Franciscan Saint Francis Health). He served as the chief of the medical staff at Saint Francis Hospital and University Heights Hospital (present-day Community South Hospital). De Wester died in April 2010.

This episode was given by De Wester's son, Jeff, who is also a family doctor.

My father told a story about a particular house call he once made. He got a call from a family that wanted him to come over as soon as possible and check on Grandma. She appeared to be very ill.

"We think Grandma's had a stroke," they told him when he arrived at their house. "She's acting really strangely, like nothing we've seen

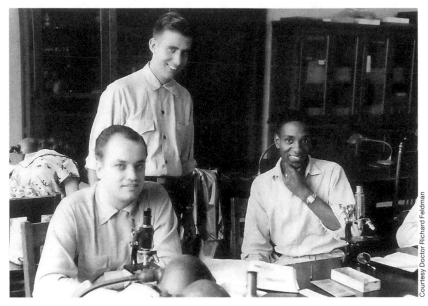

Courtesy Doctor Richard Feldman

Gerald De Wester (seated, left)

before. We don't know what is wrong with her, and we don't know what to do, doctor."

"Okay," Dad said. And he goes upstairs to check on her.

A few minutes later he calls the oldest members of the family upstairs to talk to him about his evaluation of grandma's condition. "I've got some good news and some bad news," he told them. "The good news is grandma has not had a stroke. She will be just fine by morning."

"Oh, doctor," they said, "what a relief!"

"That is certainly a relief," he replied, "but remember, I have some bad news too."

He then walks over to her bureau chest of drawers and pulls out a couple bottles of liquor. He pokes behind the curtain and comes back with another one. From under the bed, he retrieves an armful of bottles. Bottles everywhere.

"The bad news is grandma's stone cold drunk," he said.

Editor's Note: Clandestine alcohol consumption was also involved in another family doctor's amusing story that was told to the editor. "I remember one time that one of my old farmer patients fell out of a haymow and broke his hip, and they put him in the orthopedic ward at the hospital. About an hour before the scheduled surgery, I got a call to come ASAP to see him. I rushed up to the floor to see him, and when I walked in the room with the head nurse following right behind me, he threw the nurse out and had her close the door. He said, 'Now, Doc, I just have something to tell you and thought maybe it might be important. I had a stash of hooch up there in the haymow, and my wife doesn't know anything about it. I just got a little too much to drink and missed my footing and fell out of the haymow. I thought I had just better tell you in case it makes any difference to you before we go to surgery. But Doc, promise me that you won't say anything to my wife about the hooch. That would be a bigger problem than this broken hip!' I promised him it would be our secret."

78

The Godfather of Medicine

My father was known as a fearless, effective, and, at times, intimidating patient advocate. His colleagues also knew he had a robust sense of humor and loved to engage in teasing and jousting. It is not surprising that he received a nickname, "Guido, The Godfather of Medicine," for his ferocious advocacy for his patients. Defending and advocating for his patients to assure the best quality care in our complex health-care system was a mission for my father. Crossing him in this endeavor would be a mistake.

A short time after I entered practice, I became aware of this "title" and its apparent enthusiastic acceptance by many of his colleagues. I personally found the title not only appropriate, but also personally gratifying as he had publicly bestowed upon me several "titles" as a youth; these "honors" were something I would've gladly done without!

Though amused by this knowledge, I couldn't help being struck by a sense of irony in light of certain elements of my father's past. It is a well-known but quietly held truth within the De Wester family that my father's arrival in Indianapolis at the age of seventeen did not seem auspicious at the time. In fact, it was the occasion for widespread anxiety due to his socializing with various "shady" individuals, some of whom were well-known gangsters and corrupt city government officials. Hence, all the more, I was curious about his reaction to such an appellation, but was unsure if he was aware of the high honor that had been bestowed upon him. Yet only once, in the midst of discussing a patient, did I ask him if he was aware of being referred to in this way and what he thought of his "title." He looked up at me and, noting my amusement, remained silent but expressed a brief, muted smile before returning to our work.

Editor's Note: This reminiscence was provided by Jeff De Wester.

79

When Insults Are Really Expressions of Respect

As in any profession, camaraderie is an important part of medicine. Camaraderie is based on friendship, trust, admiration, and respect among colleagues. De Wester was considered an elder statesman of Indiana family medicine. Those older family doctors who successfully transcended the years with excellent clinical skills and current medical knowledge won the respect and reverence of their younger medical colleagues, both family physician and specialist.

Jeff De Wester was fortunate as a young medical student to experience that affection for his father among his colleagues. He relates the following story, an unusual expression of good-natured bantering, as an example of that admiration and respect. Seasoned, confident older doctors could hold their own in any joust. And a good contest of wits made the day that much more enjoyable.

My father was well known for many things, not the least of which was his sharp wit and love of humor. Through his interaction with family and relatives I was, of course, well acquainted with these attributes. However, prior to becoming a doctor, I knew little about how this might manifest itself in his practice of medicine. Upon entering medical training, however, it wasn't long before I became more familiar with the many facets of this wonderful part of my father's persona. In the fall of 1986 I had entered into my senior medical school electives while working at nights as an emergency department extern, both of which involved a lot of time spent at Saint Francis Hospital in Indianapolis. Thus, I entered for the first time an era of regular and enlightening interaction with many of my father's closest colleagues.

One morning, I was beginning a cardiology rotation at Saint Francis with a physician that I knew was held with the highest respect by my father. In fact, when I had solicited his advice about who I should request as a preceptor, I knew the unhesitant answer before I asked. "If you want to learn from the best in cardiology, you'll go with Buz Hickman," my father said. I knew this referred to Horace O. Hickman, MD, who my father jokingly referred to as his "adopted son." Having listened to my father on numerous occasions speak about him, I came to view my father's feelings as paternal and jokingly referred to him as dad's "adopted son." Perhaps one can appreciate why I expected an exceptional experience, although it was to be in ways I had not anticipated. Arriving at the hospital early that morning, I quickly became familiar with the odyssey that awaits the poor soul trying to locate Hickman. However, this marathon was not without merit, since it initiated my understanding of why he was called "Buz"; tracking him down was like tracking a rocket. Each time I arrived at my intended destination, the typical response was, "You just missed him."

This went on for a while until I came upon the idea of having the nursing staff inform him that I was on my way to meet him. After locating him on the fourth floor, I employed my plan and rushed onto a crowded elevator to head him off. To my surprise, the elevator doors opened on the fourth floor only to reveal an impatient-appearing Hickman, who greeted me with a loud, "You're late, wimp!"

Not sure of what to make of this unusual introductory expression of esteem, I soon realized it was just the first dose of jabs, putdowns, and sarcastic remarks that were to be administered that day. If this was my lot when studying under one of my dad's "friends," I could only wonder what would transpire interacting with an enemy.

For a couple of days my rotation continued in the same inexplicable fashion until one morning while making rounds we received a page from my father. I learned of this when Hickman approached me with, "Damn it, your old man paged me. Come on, let's see what the old gomer wants now!" In light of my ongoing confusion, I welcomed the opportunity to see them interact, and see if Hickman would serve up the same verbal cuisine to my father he'd been dishing out to me. I was not to be disappointed.

Upon meeting at the nurses' station, we sat down and to my amazement Hickman immediately launched into a verbal flurry that perhaps only a fan of boxing could fully appreciate. Situated between them, ringside, I must have been gawking as he unloaded his jabs.

"Well Guido, your son's a real daddy's boy. And what kind of crap does he have in here?" Waving my doctor bag around he exclaimed, "Hell, it must weigh twenty pounds! And what's wrong with him anyway? Every time I look around he has his head in a book; didn't he learn anything in medical school? Or was he not lucky enough to get his mother's brains?"

At around this time, I threw a glance toward the target of this assault expecting to see the equivalent of a fighter "on the ropes." On the contrary, I beheld my father relaxed, leaning slightly forward with the patronizing expression of a patient father listening to the confused ramblings of a beloved but imbecilic child. Having seen this expression before, I sat back in anticipation of his response, my feelings of irritation with Hickman already giving way to a growing sense of pity.

Like a fighter who had punched himself out, Hickman seemed to visibly slump after pausing to assess what effects had been wrought by his whirlwind, auditory barrage. Dad, looking as if encountering a bothersome flea, countered slowly and methodically, "Well, you see Buz, Jeff's not going to be a cardiologist, he's going to be a real doctor, which means he'll need REAL medical tools. He won't be able to get along with the incense and rattles that you're used to.

"And yes, I know that in your little everything's-a-nail world, it may seem that you only need a hammer, but he's going to be seeing patients with a wide variety of REAL medical problems." So, taking my bag and holding it up, Dad continued, "He needs what we call a doctor's bag." Leaning slightly farther forward, extending his hand, and speaking with the deliberate calm typical when soothing a neurotic patient he added, "And, yes, HE reads a lot; in family medicine we call that studying. Unlike you, he's going to be a primary-care doctor, which means he will be taking care of his own patients. He won't be a specialist with someone cleaning up his mistakes and carrying him like I have you all these years!"

Watching Buz during this was painful; he appeared to twitch and gasp, desperately trying to respond but only managing to flail about meaninglessly with, "Yeah but . . . well I . . . what?" Trying to maintain a straight face, a boyish grin increasingly broke through until Hickman laughed, hung his head, and put his hands up in defeat.

Standing up triumphantly, my father began to head for the elevator. "I've got a busy day Jeff, no doubt cleaning up a lot of Buz's messes, so will you please try to keep him from hurting too many more patients today?" Slowly getting up as he recovered himself, we moved out of the nurses' station with Buz mumbling, "Now you know why I've been giving you such a hard time!" As we rounded the corner out of sight, he became more animated and turned and put a finger in my face. "You have no idea what it's like! Nobody jousts with your dad and gets the better of 'em!"

I remember thinking, "Actually, I have a pretty good idea."

Later that week, I ran into Doctor Donald Lauer, one of my dad's closest friends and also a family physician. I shared my fascinating experience, naively thinking he too would be surprised. Instead, Lauer just shook his head with a look of satisfaction and as he walked away sighing, he responded, "The boy will never learn that he shouldn't try to play with the big boys."

80

A Person to Emulate

As both a resident and as the director of the family medicine residency at Saint Francis Hospital in Beech Grove/Indianapolis, the author fondly remembers the presence of De Wester staffing at the residency's outpatient clinic. He was a founding faculty member of the residency and like doctors in private practice on the Indianapolis south side, he took time away from practice and family to teach young residents in training.

For more than three decades, De Wester taught residents and students more than how to best manage a particular patient we were staffing with him. He taught them about people and about life. He shared his wisdom, his values, and his dedication to medicine. Typical of a caring family doctor with many years of experience, he was a person who possessed great insight into the human condition.

The following was shared by his son, Jeff:

The earliest memories of De Wester's children include the presence of medical students at the dinner table. Believing that the physician is inherently a teacher, it was only natural that teaching medical students and residents was one of the basic components of his medical career.

Throughout his nearly fifty years of practice he was involved as an educator, predominately through the Saint Francis Hospital Family Practice Program.

Philosophically he was convinced that the relatively recent historical separation of clinical medicine and academics was a disastrous change that had led to a severe degradation in the quality of medical education. His conviction was that clinicians should have the preeminent role as teachers of medicine to preserve real-world input into the design, direction, and execution of clinical education and medical research. Though he recognized the place of full-time academics as a part of the medical education/research team, he felt strongly that the most effective teachers of the practice of medicine were clinicians themselves.

Though he was uncomfortable with praise, he was recognized repeatedly for achievements and received numerous awards. When the Gerald M. De Wester Treatment and Research Center was opened after his death, the material contents of his practice were transferred to the new location and a search was conducted for his awards in order to place them on display. Only one could not be located—the John T. Emhardt Role Model Award. This award was given by the residents of the Saint Francis Family Medicine Residency Program to the physician that they would most want to emulate.

This award was found on display in his home library; it is the award he prized the most and the only one that he cared to place in his home after he retired.

81

A Child Found

John Records, MD, was born on January 20, 1936, and graduated from Indiana University in 1958 with a bachelor of science degree. He then continued his education at the IU School of Medicine, earning his medical degree in 1961.

Records entered practice in 1962 as a solo physician in Franklin, Indiana. Over the course of his long and dedicated career, Records practiced the wide gamut of family medicine, delivering 1,800 babies, conducting minor office surgery, and caring for pediatric and adult patients. Although planning his retirement (at least according to his wife, Pamela), he continues his private practice in Franklin.

Family physicians are consulted by phone all the time. When on call, they naturally receive some calls from people in distress. But early in his career, Records got a call he has never forgotten.

The son of a general practitioner, Records says he learned the art of medicine from his dad. He saw his father's work and decided that he was going to become a family doctor, too. He was twelve years old.

Records estimates that 40 percent of his 1961 graduating class went

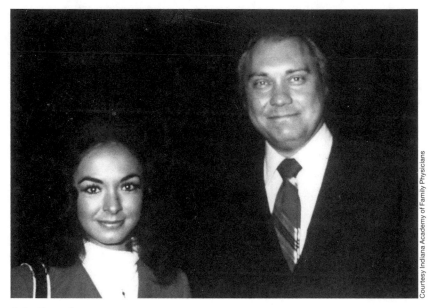

John Records

into family practice. "At our forty-fifth reunion, there was still half of the class practicing medicine," he said. "That, to me, indicates that we're either poor financial planners or that we're getting fulfillment out of what we're doing, and we want to keep doing it."

"Dad said to me, 'If you're well-schooled, you'll know what to do when you see the patient,'" Records said. "That's one of the things I have always carried with me and have never forgotten." But the elder Records also taught his son the importance of knowing one's patients. Treat them like family. It proved to be an important lesson.

One evening, while he and his wife were enjoying a night at the symphony, Records received an emergency call from the Johnson County Coroner. The call was about a family that had been killed in a terrible automobile accident. A pill bottle in the pocket of the father had Records name on it. The coroner needed him to come down and identify the bodies.

The coroner, Harley Palmer, was friend of Records. It was a somber moment as he entered the morgue. "I'll be darned, I go into the morgue and there are five bodies in there," Records recalled. "I see three kids and a husband and wife. I knew them all and identified them. They had gone across an unmarked train crossing down in Amity. They had not seen the train, and the train hit them."

Records goes on to describe the grisly scene: "It just mangled the car unmercifully. They were all killed instantly and cut up and everything. The blunt force trauma broke their necks or fractured their skulls. They were laying there just as peaceful as could be." But wait a minute. Somebody was missing. Records asked, "Where's Jennifer?'"

Investigators were unaware of a fourth child. But Records knew the entire family and told Palmer that the youngest girl was missing. Police and emergency crews picked up the bodies that were thrown from the car and extracted a couple of bodies from the wreck. But there was no sign of a five-year-old girl.

"They'd hauled the car off already," Records said, "and the little kid was down underneath the dashboard, crushed, but still living." The preschooler survived with just a broken arm. Emergency crews missed her because she was unconscious, and they didn't notice her.

"I still see her today," said Records.

82

Flames

Robert Mouser, MD, was born on October 21, 1931. He graduated early from Shortridge High School in Indianapolis, Indiana, enabling him to obtain an associate degree from Laval University in Quebec City, Quebec, before attending Wabash College. He graduated from Wabash with a degree in astronomy and history and attended the Indiana University School of Medicine, graduating in 1954. Mouser was in group practice in Indianapolis from 1957 to 1984.

Of his many accomplishments, one of the most notable is that Mouser gave the first shot of human insulin in the world for Eli Lilly and Company. Mouser died July 22, 2013.

Mouser entered medical school at the age of seventeen. He became the youngest graduate of the Indiana University School of Medicine. The Indiana General Assembly had to pass a law so he could have a medical license before the age of twenty-one. He practiced for fifty-four years until retiring in January 2008.

In addition to his private family medicine practice, Mouser was also a medical officer at the Indianapolis Motor Speedway for thirty years.

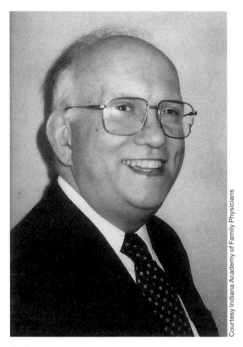

Courtesy Indiana Academy of Family Physicians

Robert Mouser

Mouser was on duty in 1964 when the race was marred by a horrific crash that involved racecar drivers Eddie Sachs and Dave McDonald, who swerved out of control and back-ended an inside wall. The car burst into flames, gathering up Sachs in the ensuing inferno. Sachs was killed instantly, but Mc-Donald survived the initial impact and fire. Mouser performed a tracheotomy on McDonald, giving him four extra hours of life. He was able to speak with his wife before he died.

With the help of Speedway physician Tom Hanna, Mouser helped revolutionize driver safety by promoting the use of Nomex fire retardant threads. At first, none of the drivers wanted to use it, but Mouser said he was able to convince a young A. J. Foyt.

"I talked to A. J. and I said, 'You know you can keep from burning your hands and arms like you had by wearing the Nomex.' He said, 'I can, Doc?' And I said yes. He decided to give it a try."

"It was a good decision. Foyt got into a fire the next year using Nomex and after that everybody used Nomex."

83

Dispensing Pills

In 1957 Mouser began his Indianapolis practice. Mouser and many doctors during that time dispensed medications, mostly inexpensive ones, to patients in his office.

"The pill-rolling companies would come by and sell you stuff. You could buy some types of medications for ninety-three cents a thousand," Mouser said. "They had twenty-six kinds of aspirin. One woman used white pills with blue polka dots on it. She had insomnia and it was the only thing that worked to make her sleep. I charged a dollar for a box full of them."

On one occasion, a doctor in another practice signed out to Mouser. He received a call from one of this doctor's female patients whom he was totally unfamiliar with. "She said, 'I've run out of my pills, can you get me some more?'" Mouser said.

Mouser told the patient he wasn't sure, but asked her to describe what the pills looked like. Hoping to find a clue in identifying the drug from the name of the manufacturer, Mouser asked the patient to read any markings on the side. She couldn't pronounce it, but she told him that the markings were p-l-a-c-e-b-o.

84

Bantering with the Sister

Bernard Emkes, MD, Mouser's former practice partner, related his favorite story to the author. For those who knew Mouser, it seems characteristic of his personality:

Many, many years ago, Mouser was a member of a committee that developed a new set of patient chart forms for use at some Indianapolis hospitals including Saint Vincent Hospital in Indianapolis. The committee's work was done and the forms were ready for final approval by each hospital. Mouser decided to drop the forms off at Saint Vincent one morning before he made his hospital rounds.

Back then, as in most hospitals, there was a large panel of physicians' names on the wall near the doctors' entrance to the hospital. Each name had a little light switch the physician would flip on when entering the hospital. By viewing the lighted name, hospital staff and operators would know that the physician was in the hospital. Near that panel was the office of the sister who had the responsibility for the approval of the medical forms. Entering the office, he found that the sister wasn't there, so he placed the pile of forms on her desk and proceeded to the wards.

Mouser and this sister had a great relationship; both possessed a lively sense of humor and they loved to banter back and forth. Mouser chose to leave a particular form in the pile that was really meant only for use at another hospital. The form: consent for elective abortion.

As was the custom, when leaving the hospital doctors would flip their name light to off. With his rounds completed and ready to depart the hospital, Mouser searched the panel to locate his name to turn off his light.

His name was gone.

85

A Stranger in Need

James Ray, MD, was born on March 3, 1939, and was raised in Bloomington, Indiana. After graduating with honors from the Indiana University School of Business in 1963, he left Bloomington to attend the IU School of Medicine, graduating in 1968. Ray began practicing in 1969 after completing an internal medicine internship at the IU Medical Center in Indianapolis.

Ray was a solo practitioner in family medicine for more than thirty-five years in Bloomington. In 1992 he was elected as chief of staff at Bloomington Hospital. He also received a faculty appointment in the Department of Family Medicine at the IU School of Medicine as a volunteer clinical assistant professor. Ray served his country as a member of the Indiana National Guard.

Ray was recognized as the Family Physician of the Year in 1992 by the Indiana Academy of Family Physicians. He retired from practice in 2004 and continued his involvement in medicine by volunteering at the Volunteers in Medicine Clinic in Bloomington. He continues to reside in Bloomington with his wife of fifty-two years, Donna. Ray has been active in the First Christian Church for many years as a moderator, elder, and teacher.

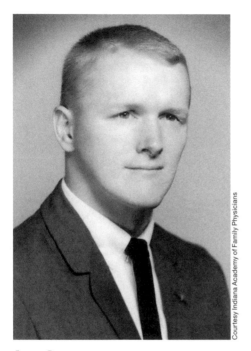

Courtesy Indiana Academy of Family Physicians

James Ray

Ray was the type of doctor who always took his patients' calls, no matter what time of the day or night. Some calls even came in as late as two o'clock in the morning. Beyond holding traditional office hours, Ray operated on his patients' schedules. His wife and former office manager, Donna, recalled, "When the girls would apply for a position they would say 'what time do you start?' and 'what time do you finish?' I would tell them quitting time is just whenever we finish. If somebody came home from work and found their kids sick and needed to bring them in after 5:00 p.m., the answer was always yes."

In Ray's office, if a patient called during the day with a question about test results, a prescription, or whether they should make an appointment, the doctor and his staff recorded every call and made sure to call back every patient personally at the end of the day. And Ray always called back any abnormal test results himself. "If the office phone rang a real person answered it," Donna added. "We didn't use machines to answer the phones."

There were hardly any computers used at Ray's office, even later in his career when they were readily available. For taking down notes during patient consultations, Ray preferred to use a tape recorder instead of a computer, so that he could keep eye contact with the patient. In short, Ray's office was always personal.

"We told our employees, 'it's a family practice office and that's how we want to treat everyone,'" said Donna. "We treated our employees as family, and we treated every patient as a family member and as someone who we respected."

This sense of family and of taking extra time out of his day to care for others did not extend only to Ray's patients. He remembered a time he and his family were on vacation and he was called upon to help a complete stranger: "We were walking through a parking lot up in the Smoky Mountains looking at a vista quite a few years ago. It was I, my wife, and our three boys there. We had no medical supplies with us because we were on vacation. Out of the blue, my oldest son spotted a man alone in his car and said, 'Dad, this person looks like he's not breathing!'

"So I walked over to the car and, sure enough, the man inside actually wasn't breathing. There was a park ranger there, but he wasn't really doing much. Somebody had to help this man. So, I got the man out of the car and gave him mouth-to-mouth right there on the ground in the parking lot. We called an ambulance then and they took him to the hospital. He survived and did fine.

"Afterwards I started wondering, 'What if that guy was sick? What if I caught something from him?' I called the hospital and the man had signed out, but I eventually got a hold of his family doctor and found out that everything was fine; I hadn't contracted any disease from him. I was worried afterwards, sure, but what was I supposed to do? It was a crucial situation; the man was not breathing and needed help.

"I think things are different for people, including doctors, these days. I think some doctors would be reluctant to do mouth-to-mouth on a total stranger in that situation, not knowing what their health history is. But I just did what I had to do. It was part of the philosophy of medicine in the old days that when someone needs help, you help them. And you ask questions later. "I will always remember that day; my kids thought I was a hero."

86

The Invisible Baby

Ray did a little of everything. He enjoyed cardiology, but has always been happy with his choice of family medicine because it gave him a chance to practice many different kinds of medicine and to help people in many different kinds of situations.

He remembers one situation, in particular, that cannot be described any way other than different:

In 1969 I had come back from medical school, which I attended in Indianapolis, to Bloomington, where I settled and founded my practice. The very first baby I delivered was that year, and it was a truly unforgettable experience.

I got a call from a woman saying that her daughter was pregnant and was going into labor. She sounded confused and sort of shaken up on the phone, but I chalked it up to the typical jitters associated with a first baby. So when I got the call, I sent the girl to the hospital and met her and her mother there. I delivered the baby, and both the baby and the new mother were healthy and happy. I was surprised, though, when I found out that the young woman hadn't received any prenatal care whatsoever. In fact, her mother didn't even know she was pregnant until the contractions started, and the baby was already coming! The night of the delivery was the first this girl's mother had ever heard of the baby, and that's when she called me.

Once I got a good look at the daughter I realized why she had been able to hide her pregnancy from her mother throughout the entire nine months: she must have weighed more than two hundred pounds!

But, a mother's love can be blinding. After the baby was delivered and all was said and done, the girl's mother pulled me aside and whispered to me, "I just don't understand how this got past me, doctor. She's always been such a puny girl!"

87

Outdoor Obstetrics

Marvin Christie, MD, was born on September 19, 1930, and grew up on the south side of Indianapolis, Indiana. He attended Southport High School before attending Indiana University, Bloomington, receiving his bachelor of science in anatomy and physiology in 1952. He graduated from the IU School of Medicine in 1955. Christie completed his internship with the U.S. Air Force at Letterman Hospital in San Francisco, California, in 1956. He was honorably discharged in June 1958. Christie worked in the Beech Grove/Indianapolis area in a partnership for twenty years before moving into group practice. He delivered about 1,500 babies, he also performed procedures including tonsillectomies, adenoidectomies, and myringotomies for thirty years.

He has been medical staff president of University Heights Hospital (now part of Community Health Network) and Saint Francis Hospital. Although he retired from active family practice in 1988, he still works for the Federal Aviation Administration as an aviation medical examiner.

Christie likes to tell his patients he was born before the "Star Spangled Banner" was our national anthem. It is true. The national anthem was officially designated by an act of Congress in 1931.

In college Christie played basketball for Coach Branch McCracken at Indiana University. His studies forced him to quit the team. His teammate, Frank O'Bannon, spent all of his time sitting on the bench. O'Bannon did better in politics, becoming governor of Indiana in 1997. "I was fortunate and went right through med school—three years of pre-med school and four years of medical school and three years of military," Christie remembered.

According to Christie, family doctors did a little bit of everything, including tonsillectomies. "Back in those days, if you could demonstrate your ability, then you didn't need any residency training," he said. Obstetrics was also part of his general practice.

In 1954 Christie was a junior in medical school. He had a straight-eight 1938 Oldsmobile coupe that he bought from classmate Mort Willcutts for sixty-five dollars. It was his ticket to a unique program that no longer exists at the IU School of Medicine. He would deliver babies in Indianapolis disadvantaged neighborhoods. They called it "outdoor OB."

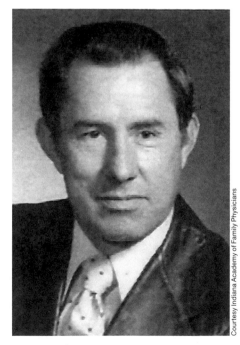

Marvin Christie

Courtesy Indiana Academy of Family Physicians

It was an unusual program that called for junior medical students to do home deliveries. For many medical students, it was a first-time experience. Christie related the time that one student was bewildered by a gray protrusion from an expectant mother's vagina.

"It didn't look like a baby's head," Christie recalled. "It didn't look like a baby's head, so he started scraping it. Of course, it was the bag of water." Christie indicates that the scraping caused the bag to explode spraying the young medical student with fluid.

"We'd go out in the home and you had to stay there," Christie said. "You'd get out there and maybe she wouldn't deliver for twelve hours." The program was a trial by fire for medical students. Armed with only a medical bag and forceps, they would spend hours awaiting for a delivery. Christie said many of his mothers and fathers resisted going to the hospital. As he explained it, there were some myths and superstitions about having babies in a hospital where certain germs would flourish and people died. Students could only call for an ambulance for a good reason.

Christie remembered one time when the father became agitated during the labor. The last time his wife had delivered, the baby died. Christie then decided to call the ambulance, but had to walk down the street to a local tavern because the house didn't have a telephone.

Interestingly, several babies that year were named Marvin. Christie said after the delivery, he would be filling out the birth certificate. "I'd say, 'What's his name?'" Christie said. "She'd say, 'What's your name doctor?'" He'd try to talk them out of it, but several babies born in Indianapolis in 1954 were named Marvin.

That was the last semester that IU provided the neighborhood OB program. Christie said the university attorneys started to become concerned and malpractice was starting to gain traction. "In all honesty, they were sending unqualified people—not even licensed—out into the home," he said.

Christie went on to deliver babies in his private practice. "Obstetrics is a pleasant practice, but the tragedies can be absolutely overwhelming," he recalled. "I was fortunate. I didn't have any problems at all out there delivering babies." He charged thirty dollars for delivering an infant in 1958. That included all of the prenatal visits and the delivery. When he wanted to increase it to fifty dollars five years later, he argued with his partner, Doctor Charles Dill, who believed that the increase would cost them their entire business. Up through the 1970s, when he quit obstetrics, Christie only charged a hundred and fifty dollars!

88

A Cautionary Tale

Christie recalls his first year of medical school in Bloomington and the plight of one unfortunate student.

It was the first day of class and Christie was sitting in an auditorium amongst his peers feeling dumber than them. "Everybody looked smarter than you," he laughed. "I felt like I was the dumbest guy in there. You know how that is. You know you're in there with a bunch of guys that are good students.

"If you could survive that first year, you pretty well knew you were going to graduate. But that first year was the tough one to get out of. There were a lot of summer repeat courses, mainly physiology. A lot of guys were just kicked out period."

Nevertheless, it was the first day of medical school and the dean of the IU School of Medicine, John Van Nuys, addressed the students. The stage was littered with the professors of anatomy and physiology. "Dean Van Nuys asked the students to congratulate a particular student and said, 'I want you to congratulate Walter Daly, the number one scholastic choice from the state of Indiana,'" Christie recounted. "He said, 'Walt, come down here.' And Walt came down. In other words, he was the smartest guy in that class."

"Then he said, 'Now, I want to introduce the number one student from out of state, Mr. Paul Watson from Manhattan University in New York.' And everybody clapped. Van Nuys gets down there and he puts his arm around Watson and he said, 'I also want to tell you that Mr. Watson is a Goddamn fraud!' He said, 'He manufactured all of his own transcripts. He never went to Manhattan.' And he kept squeezing him tighter. 'Everything he's done has been a fraud. He hasn't even had any pre-med. All these documents that were unbelievably good.' Then he said, 'Security, would you take Mr. Watson? We'll talk to you later Mr. Watson.'"

It made quite an impression on the young students who were unsure of what to do next. "I thought, 'My God, if they mention my name, I'm dead!'" Christie said. "So then Van Nuys said, 'That will be all for today!' We've often wondered what happened to Mr. Paul Watson."

89

A Grateful Cat

Ross Egger, MD, was born on March 24, 1937, and was raised in North Liberty, Indiana, in Saint Joseph County. He received his bachelor of science degree in biology and chemistry from Ball State University in 1959. He then attended the Indiana University School of Medicine, graduating in 1962. After completing his internship, Egger entered practice in July 1963.

For most of his career, Egger worked as a solo physician. His scope included obstetrics and inpatient hospital work. In addition to his clinical work, Egger also served in various positions in the health insurance industry and served for years as the director of the Family Medicine Residency Program at Ball Memorial Hospital in Muncie, Indiana. He was an adjunct professor at Ball State University and received a faculty appointment in the Department of Family Medicine at the IU School of Medicine as a volunteer clinical associate professor.

He was honored by the American Academy of Family Physicians with the prestigious Thomas W. Johnson Award for career contributions to family medicine education in 1979 and served as president of the Indiana Academy of Family Physicians from 1974 to 1975. As a family physician, Egger treated whole families. In this case he really treated the whole family:

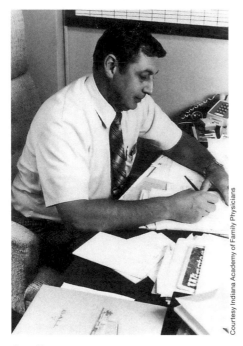

Courtesy Indiana Academy of Family Physicians

Ross Egger

I'll never forget my very first house call, because it provided another first for me. A lady called me and told me she thought her son had pneumonia. I told her not to worry, and that I would come by right after office hours that day.

That's what I did: I got in my car and went to this lady's house, and, sure enough, her son had pneumonia. By the way, most patients are right about their children, and especially back in those days. Most patients were correct about what their children had because they knew what to expect from their own childhood experiences with diseases.

So, I gave her son a shot of penicillin and started to pack my doctor's bag to get ready to leave. But before I had a chance to start making my way downstairs to leave, she asked me a question.

"By the way, doc, do cats get pneumonia?"

And I said, "Yeah, well matter of fact I think they do."

"Well, could you check my cat?" she asked.

Now I was by no means trained with any sort of veterinary care, but I felt it was my responsibility to help this patient as best I could. "I guess I could take a look," I said. "I know where the lungs are, at least."

So I took my stethoscope to this kitty cat's chest—he was good and held still, which I was thankful for—and it did sound to me like he had pneumonia. I told the lady that's what it sounded like and she looked at me, and then at her cat, and then back to me again. She scratched her head. "Well, could you give him penicillin shot too?"

So I did some calculations and figured out the dose that I should give the cat. I gave the cat a shot in the butt and she told me later that her cat got better! So, I cured her son and cured the cat, too. That's the only time that happened to me, and it was on my first ever house call. Quite a way to learn about people's lives, that's for sure.

90

A Cure Worse Than the Disease

Egger remembers an unusual case:

One of my most memorable patients was a woman in her mid-forties who came in to see me experiencing the classic symptoms of hyperthyroidism, which essentially means an overactive thyroid. She was experiencing weight loss, a rapid pulse, and she was sweaty and hot all the time. She also reported difficulty sleeping. I spoke with her about her symptoms and listened to her, and we did three or four thyroid tests that all came back normal, including a radioactive iodine test.

It was unbelievable to me that all these tests came back negative. "This is impossible," I said. "You have hyperthyroidism. I just know it."

Finally, the fourth test we took came back positive for hyperthyroidism. This search-and-find routine went on for a year. That is one of the main differences about family practice docs of my generation versus many of the docs today. Today more emphasis is put on taking tests, and test results. With this patient, and many others like her, I relied on my intuition and on paying attention to her symptoms and listening to her.

Eventually, with persistence, we did find the hyperthyroidism in this patient. We operated on her and removed a thyroid nodule that we found. As a result of the procedure she calmed down, got back up to a healthy weight, and just felt perfect. All was well.

Well, one day a couple months later she came into my office with some new problems she was experiencing. "I can't get anything done!" she said, "Could I have my hyperthyroidism back?!"

We had a good laugh about that. She was used to working something like twelve to fourteen hours a day in the home, and not sleeping. She could just go, go, go. So she wanted to have her hyperthyroidism back again. I'm not sorry to say I had to deny that request!

Editor's Note: I am reminded of a patient who also presented with obvious hyperthyroidism. He was a young athletic man who was a tennis player. He was distraught both with the diagnosis and the treatment plan of radioactive iodine to ablate his gland. Why? Since he developed the symptoms of hyperthyroidism he was playing his best game ever, and he was reluctant to give up his condition. But he did go through with the treatment after it was explained how important it ultimately was to his health. Unfortunately, his tennis game suffered a setback after he was treated, just as he suspected it would!

91

A Special Prescription

Possessing a good sense of humor and knowing when to use it is part of the art of medicine, as in Egger's following story:

One of my more interesting patients was a pretty ornery older farmer I had a really fun relationship with. We would joke back and forth a lot but also he knew that he could trust me to take care of him.

Well, he came into my office one day and I asked how everything was going for him.

"Pretty good," he said, "but I'll tell you, what I really need is a prescription for sex."

I said, "You're eighty years old!"

He said, "Well, that's what I need. I don't need any of this other stuff." What are you going to do? There was no arguing with this guy, and anyway it was just fun. So I wrote him out an actual prescription on my official pad for exactly what he requested. He took it home, and the next day I got a call back from his wife. "Just what drugstore do you think he's going to go to, to get this filled, doc?" We had a good laugh. That's what our relationship was like.

92

The Urine Sample

An odd little moment for Egger:

One of the best ways to find out whether a patient has a urinary infection is to obtain a urine sample. As is still the case, patients had the option of taking the test right there in our office or taking it at home and bringing it in to us. In either instance, we provided the receptacle for collecting the urine.

Well, one lady, I don't know what happened. I guess she lost her little receptacle we'd given her, and she brought in her urine specimen in a perfume bottle! Now, it does take quite an imagination to figure out how in the world somebody could get urine into a bottle that's got an opening in the top of maybe two millimeters. We had to shake it out just to test it.

That was really odd, I thought. You know, we should have asked her how she did it.

93

Better than Money

Many older family physicians remember the time when they were frequently paid by their patients in ways other than by check, cash, or credit card. Sometimes the alternative payments and the little gifts that docs received from their patients were expressions of affection and appreciation. It was a simpler and more personalized time, as Egger reminisces:

One of the first things you had to understand as a family doctor was that you wouldn't always get paid. Now, that's not as crummy as it sounds. Sure, sometimes it meant you just simply didn't get paid. That was one thing that has definitely changed over the years. Back when I first started practicing in the 1960s, if patients came in and didn't feel that the service I gave them was appropriate or helpful, they just wouldn't pay me. That was a fun part about medicine and the part that intrigued me most—how honest patients were. The times when they didn't pay me, well I thought in a way that was very fair, and it let you know pretty quickly whether you were providing what the patients wanted.

At other times "not getting paid" just meant not being paid in dollars and cents. What I got from the patients in lieu of money some-times was much more valuable. Ladies, for example, would bring in all kinds of baked goods. An office visit cost only three dollars back when I first started, so a little bundle of baked goods would be a very fair trade and it made me so happy.

I loved that. Things were extra special when holiday time came around. Patients would bring fruit baskets and homemade goods and crafts. A lot of times they'd bring it in lieu of pay, or as an extra thank-you if they knew I had taken a lot longer than normal on an office visit with them, or maybe I made one more visit to their home that I didn't charge them for.

It seemed like whatever I did for my patients, it would always come back to me in double. They would bring coupons for a free meal at a restaurant. Coupons had just gotten started back then, but I remember a couple patients brought those, and that was really special. Eating out at a restaurant was a real treat.

For some people, it became part of a routine. In a way, it was like becoming a member of the family once you made a couple house calls. I had one patient, a little old lady I'll never forget. She was about sev-enty-eight or eighty years old and lived by herself; her husband had died years before. She lived on a beautiful farm that her husband had homesteaded, actually. And oh, they had all kinds of fruits and vegeta-bles, and it was just lovely and abundant out there.

I made house calls once a month for her—she required that I would stop by at about 7:00 a.m., and she would have the biggest breakfast I'd ever seen in my life waiting for me. Every month. There would be homemade sausages, berries, eggs, just everything. That was the deal, developed by her of course. I would stop by and have breakfast, and she would tell me how she felt. She was very pleased with that.

And there was one guy; I'll never forget him either. He gave us hay for a long, long time. We had two ponies back then, and he helped me very much. This fellow, every time he came for a doctor visit he paid in hay. I think he came in twice a year, and he would ask me how my hay was. I would say, "Aw, I could use some." And he would tell me he'd have it out there tomorrow. That was great, I thought. Especially because—believe it or not—hay was worth more than my office visit was! Hay was about four dollars or five dollars a bale, so I was getting a great deal. It sure was different back then.

94
Susan

Jack Higgins, MD, was born on July 12, 1936. He served in the U.S. Navy from 1954 until 1957. After his military service, he attended Indiana University, where he received his bachelor of arts degree in 1961 before continuing his education at the IU School of Medicine, graduating in 1964. He completed an internship at Marion County General Hospital in 1965 and subsequently entered practice in Kokomo, Indiana, where he was raised. For thirty-three years he worked as a solo physician until he transitioned into hospital work for the remaining seven years of his career.

Indiana governor Joseph Kernan awarded Higgins the Sagamore of the Wabash award. He has also received two of the Indiana Academy of Family Physicians' awards—the Lester D. Bibler award for his many contributions to Indiana family medicine, as well as being selected Family Physician of the Year. Higgins retired from practice in January 2005.

Higgins provides us in the following story a simple fact—sometimes patients come to the doctor for reasons other than the usual medical care.

A very popular physician had died in July of the year I began my practice. Almost all his patients transitioned to me, so that I saw about

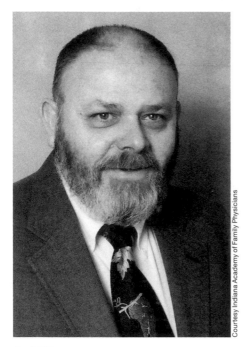

Courtesy Indiana Academy of Family Physicians

Jack Higgins

thirty patients on my very first day practicing!

There was one I remember who had been a patient of this doctor. She was slightly mentally disturbed, and she had been getting estrogen shots in one arm and B-12 shots in the other arm, once a week, for twenty years. Her arms were just like wood. You could just build a desk with her arms, that's what they felt like. Her name was Susan.

Obviously I wanted to wean this woman off her shots, so when she came in, I suggested she wait two weeks before coming back this time, instead of one. "Do you think I can go that long?" Susan said. She looked worried, and I could tell she was nervous.

I told her it would be okay and to trust me.

Going to the doctor was her social event. She would get all dressed up and gussied up for it. So you can imagine my surprise when she came back two weeks later. I don't think she'd even changed her clothes. "I just can't go two weeks without my shots," she pled.

So, I go back to a week and keep trying to stretch her out to wait longer, but after several months I finally just gave up. Even if her body didn't need the shots, she needed the shots to stay mentally stable. After that I saw her as the first patient every Monday afternoon for three or four years. It was hard to see her, but I had to.

One day I was about two hours late coming into the office, and I was in a big hurry. It was Monday afternoon, so Susan was there, as always. I hurriedly set to work on her; I was eager to just be done with her. I put a blood pressure cuff on her arm, and I'm not even sure I listened to her heart. I just pumped it up and put it down. I gave her the shots, one in each arm, told her she was doing well and that I'd see her next week.

I headed for the door and reached for the doorknob, and then I heard her say, "Dr. Higgins?" in a small voice.

"What, Susan?"

She said, "When my last doctor died, I didn't think I'd ever find anybody to replace him. But, he never spent as much time with me as you do."

I just turned right around and sat down and talked to her for about a half an hour. Most days when she came in I did sit and talk with her for a few minutes, but that day I'd already been feeling a little guilty for being late, and then she put that on me. I just had to sit down and have a chat. It was the only thing I could do. It was, of course, the right thing for a doctor to do.

95

The Thrill of It All

Higgins had particular critical care and emergency surgical aspects to his family medicine career. He enjoyed treating the sickest of the sick the most. As he explains, these were exciting times:

When I worked as a family doctor I scrubbed in for a bunch of surgeries at the hospital in town. I scrubbed just about every day, for something or other. All of the surgeons at that time were solo doctors, and they were always looking for help. I was quick to volunteer because I loved the energy.

Don't get me wrong—I loved my patients in the office, but the stuff at the hospital, it just seemed like you accomplished more. I loved that. Sometimes in the office it was, honestly, just a lot of reassuring people that there wasn't anything seriously wrong with them!

In general, I like sick people. I enjoyed doing a lot of intensive-care work because it made me feel like I was really making a difference in people's lives. That's one of the big differences I see between docs nowadays and the way it was in the golden age of family medicine, when I began practicing. Docs today don't want to take care of everybody who is sick. They just want to triage them and order some tests and send them to somebody else. I could never understand that.

Me? I grew up taking care of everything. I can't do invasive cardiology and things like that, but I think I can take care of most people in heart failure, and I can take care of heart problems as well as most cardiologists can. That's just how things were back then—the family doctor did it all. You didn't send your patients away to a specialist, a stranger, unless you really needed to.

Working in the ER and working on critical patients just gave me such a sense of accomplishment. I love making people better. To see somebody who is dying one day and better the next day is just the most rewarding thing there is. And to know that it was me who helped make the person better—that's what I live for.

When I was young and strong I could hold retractors, and I liked to do it, so I ended up on a lot of surgeries helping out that way—the surgeon would do his side and I would do mine. I was on call seven days a week for thirty-three years. I couldn't get enough.

We did some exciting surgeries. We used to do a lot of trauma and a lot of car wrecks. Fight wounds and gunshots, too. Working those surgeries are all kind of heroic feeling. I'll never forget Friday nights at the ER. We used to call it the "Friday night knife and gun club." Guys would go out and get drunk and start fighting. You'd always get somebody coming in with a knife wound or a gunshot wound or something.

When patients like that came in, you just had to act fast. I would be called in, and I would have to dive right in. Literally, in some cases. There were a number of instances where I had had my hand in a belly without gloves on. There would be a ruptured aortic aneurysm or something. The patient would come in, and the surgeon would call me. I would get there, and immediately he would have me grab a hold of the aorta so he could go scrub. After he scrubbed, I would go scrub. You couldn't do that today, no way.

We used to do a lot of things barehanded, back then. We never thought much about it, just had to act quickly in the moment. If somebody was bleeding during a procedure you never thought about putting your gloves on, you just mashed on it!

We always tried to scrub before opening a belly, but a couple times things were just bleeding so bad we had to stop it first and then scrub. Obviously, stopping the bleeding was our first priority. When I first started AIDS wasn't around. When it came around, we all started being a little more cautious. Nowadays, it isn't common to even sew up cuts without gloves.

Sometimes, as a matter of fact, gloves can even be a detriment. I am proud to say I have had my finger in a number of hearts in my day, and I remember sticking a finger in a patient's heart once in the ER to plug a hole from a knife wound. I was plugging while the surgeon was sewing up the wound around my finger. And wouldn't you know it? He caught the edge of the rubber glove and sewed my finger right in there!

96

The Ones That Didn't Make It

Family physicians experience both the joys and sorrows of treating their patients. Bringing a new life into the world is one of the most heartwarming and humbling experiences that can be found in medicine. But Higgins understands that nature has its ways, and that this miracle does not always come about as one hopes. And when it does not, it is an exceedingly sad time for both the family and the doctor:

I delivered many babies in my time as a family practice doc. Most of the time, it was a happy and rewarding experience. You deliver the baby, and then you get to follow the kids as they grow up and accomplish their goals. It's hard to describe. It's just something that you don't get in any other profession. Every time I delivered a baby I got chills. It is just a miracle.

But part of it, unfortunately, is that there are disappointments and heartbreaks, times of staggering sadness. Occasionally, I had a bad thing happen. One of my saddest times as a family physician was when I had a set of triplets. It was probably just two or three years after I came to town. All of the babies were about three pounds each and they just

. . . they should have survived. If it had been today, those babies would have survived. Without question. As it was, only one of them made it. We lost two of the three because of severe respiratory distress and prematurity of the lungs. That's still one of my most regrettable cases, looking back.

I was so desperate to save them, but I couldn't. I put all three babies on a ventilator knowing it wouldn't work. I just had to try. Nobody had ever really done that before in town that I knew of. I remember I also put umbilical catheters in the babies to help stabilize and support them, which had never been done before at Kokomo. I called Riley Hospital, and they didn't have anything else to offer. It was a very sad night.

I still feel terribly about those babies. Today, it would have been so easy. With the ventilators we have and the techniques we use today, they would have lived. You have medicine now that helps mature the lungs, and it's just a sad thing to think back. Three pounds. They weren't little tiny one pound babies that today may even make it.

Everything changes. The mother of those triplets was a nurse. I followed that baby, the one that made it, and gave him special attention all his life. She had him, at least.

Everybody always asks me how many babies I delivered, and I never know what to tell them. I always thought the one I was delivering was the one that counted. I don't know how many I delivered, really. I just enjoyed each one. I enjoyed watching the kids grow up very, very much. And I also remember the ones that didn't.

97

Come Sleet or Come Snow

Gene Ress, MD, was born on January 4, 1935, in Tell City, Indiana. He attended Indiana University, obtaining his undergraduate degree in 1956 and his medical degree at the IU School of Medicine in 1960. Ress completed an internship at Saint Mary's Hospital in Evansville, Indiana, before beginning private practice in 1961.

He began in a group practice before changing to a solo practice. He worked with the U.S. Army as a physician from 1962 to 1963. Ress continues to practice today in Tell City, where he was named "Distinguished Citizen" in 2000.

Ress recalls an era when doctors really pulled together. There was less concern about taking care of just your own practice. There was a sense of community. It was a wonderful time of camaraderie:

In 1978 there was a blizzard here in Tell City. Just before I was getting ready to head home from a busy night at the office at midnight, I got a call from a man who lived about fifteen minutes out of town. "It's my wife," he said, "She's gonna have her baby tonight." I could hear the worry in his voice. "Can you make it to the hospital?" he pleaded.

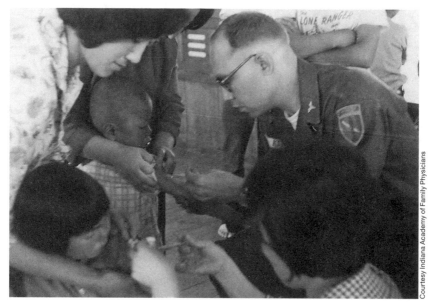

Gene Ress during his army service.

I said, "Can you make it to the hospital?" He told me they would make it. They had a truck and concrete blocks in the back.

"Well OK then," I said. "If you can make it, I can make it."

So I opened my garage, and the snow was at least two feet deep. More was coming down on top of that, and it was piling up fast. I started backing my car out a little bit at a time. I was pulling in and then revving back, and I did that over and over again. It was taking me quite a while, to say the least.

The funny thing was, I had called the police before I was going to leave and told them, "If you all are out and about and you see an old baldheaded doctor trying to get to the hospital, give him a helping hand would you?"

So I was about halfway out of my driveway and a car pulled up and honked the horn. It was a police car! And they had chains on the tires. "We'll take you, doc!" they said. So they took me up to the hospital in the police car, and I delivered the baby that night.

At that time our hospital had about fifty to sixty beds and that night they were all full. So the next morning, I told the nurses that were there from the night before to call all the doctors and tell them I'll see everybody's patients today. The snow was piling up even more; nobody could get out. So I made rounds on about fifty-five patients that morning. (I didn't have anything better to do anyway!) But that was by far the largest and the longest rounds I ever made. I'm sure one of the other doctors would have done it for me.

98

Careful What You Ask a Child!

Every family doctor can tell you about an unusual object that they removed from a child's ear. Ress had an amusing episode with a little twist:

When I opened my practice in 1961 a salesman came by to sell me my medical tools and supplies. I bought everything I needed to get started, examining tables and other important items, mostly big stuff. But before he left he held up a small item I'd never seen before. "You know, you're gonna need this," he said. He held up a little syringe. He said it was used to flush ears out.

"I've never used anything like that in medical school," I said. I told him thanks but I didn't think I needed it.

He just laughed, and told me he would give it to me, free of charge. "You'll see," he said. "You'll need it."

And sure enough, I used that little syringe on almost a daily basis. I lived in a town where there was woodworking, so it was very common to need wood and dust flushed out of ears. But honestly, all kinds of people needed their ears flushed out to get wax out and so forth. So I used warm water and used the syringe to squirt the water in, and when it hit the ear drum it would flush things out.

And I'll tell you: over the years, I squirted some very strange things out of people's ears. I remember one little girl in particular, about five or six years old. Her mother brought her in to see me and told me she thought her daughter had a grain of corn in her ear.

Sure enough, there was a fairly large corn kernel in this little girl's ear, and I've got to say, she must have been pretty talented—that corn kernel was really in there deep! It was a little uncomfortable for her getting it out, I'm sure. But we got it out with my trusty syringe, and I set the corn on the table.

We were sitting there talking—the girl's mother and me—and the mother was fussing a little bit. "Now how in the world did you do that?" she asked her daughter.

And darn it if she didn't pick up the corn and stick it right back in her ear! I had a big belly laugh. "I guess that's how she did it," I said. And I had to use my syringe to get out the same kernel a second time.

99

The Fire

Small-town people pull together in adversity. Ress remembers a time when a community rallied together for him. It is an indication of the affection, respect, and gratitude given to their family doctor:

Shortly after I built my office in Tell City, I was out of town in Louisville for a weekend with my wife and daughter. At three o'clock in the morning I got a telephone call from one of my nurses. She told me the office was on fire.

I asked her what happened, and she told me not to worry. "We've got it taken care of," she said. She told me it started in the back of the building, and while the fire was burning in the back of the building and the firemen were putting it out, she and her husband and two of my nephews were carrying all the medical charts out for me. They were carrying every last one out, and saving them. And then the word got out. People from all over town came and helped carry out my charts and made sure all the important things from my office were safe.

Something funny about this experience is that when I was in Louisville and getting the telephone call, my wife and daughter heard the phone ring and they heard me talking, but didn't know exactly what it was about. My nurse who called told me there was really nothing I could do. She said the fire-fighters got the fire put out, and they're going to stay here the rest of the night to make sure it stays out.

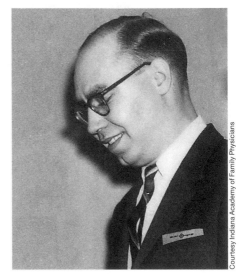

Doctor Ress

I said, "Well I think I'm just going to come down at seven in the morning in that case." And she said that would be fine. Well, I got up at 6:30 the next morning. I was getting dressed and my wife said, "It's 6:30 in the morning! Where are you going?"

I said, "I'm going home."

"Why?" She replied.

"Well, our office burned down last night." Man did I get chewed out! "Why didn't you tell me?" she demanded.

"You wouldn't have slept all night! I just decided to let you sleep, and I couldn't do anything anyway." Well, that's the worst I've ever been fussed at by my wife. She cared so much. Everybody did.

We have a furniture factory in town. After the fire a fellow came from the furniture factory to see me and said, "I'm going to get all of your furniture that's been smoked and we're going to take it down to my place, and I'm going to refinish it all." I was just taken aback. "Can you do that?" He said of course he could. I told him I would be so grateful, and I would arrange to pick up everything. He wouldn't hear it. "No, we're going to take care of everything," he said.

For the equipment in my office that had gotten all smoky in the fire, my staff and three or four other couples came and got it all out and cleaned it up until it was good as new.

Well, that fellow that did the entire office furniture repair wouldn't take a dime. And all these people volunteered cleaning all the instruments and getting everything together. They actually went through my charts that were smoked and made copies so they wouldn't smell.

I was so filled with joy and gratitude. I took fifty people to the dinner theater in New Albany to thank all of them, and we had such a lovely, memorable evening. Of course, the goodwill was just miraculous; there's just nothing you can do to thank people. This is the way people are.

Small towns are wonderful. Most people are wonderful. It's a great life being a family practice doctor. If you just allow it to happen.

100

Doing What Needs to Be Done

Ress gives us an example of a simpler time in medicine, when doctors had fewer options and resources and had less hesitation to do what needed to be done, sometimes knowing that the best course of action was not the optimal thing to do.

When I was an intern, one of the family doctors I worked under used to sit and talk with me and give me advice. We talked a lot, even after work, after hours. Sometimes I wouldn't know exactly what he was talking about, but then his lessons would bubble up later in my career, when I was in a situation. "Oh, that's what he meant by that." I would think. All through the years I thought that at various times. This story is about one of those times.

"You'll do some things you never thought you'd do," my mentor once told me. "You'll get called on a house call at 3:00 a.m. and you'll have to make do with what you've got."

Sure enough, ten years down the line I got called on a house call at 3:00 a.m. I could tell immediately that the patient really needed a shot of penicillin right away. I went into my bag and saw I only had one syringe, used. And, of course, at that time all the syringes were glass syringes that had to either be new or re-sterilized. I did not have any sterilizing equipment with me.

What did I do? Well, I thought, "This is just wrong," but I went outside and washed the sucker out with the garden hose. And I gave the patient his penicillin shot.

I did wash the syringe as much as I could, and the patient survived. He didn't get any disease from it. I was proud of what I did. I acted in the moment, and I did what I had to do. It was better to do that than not treat him at all, which is how it would be today.

Today you wouldn't dare do what I did. And, in many ways, I think that's a shame that doctors can't do what they just know needs to be done.

101

With a Little Help from My Friends

Fred Haggerty, MD, was born on February 15, 1932, in Montana, but grew up in northeastern Indiana. Before college, he served in the U.S. Air Force. He attended Indiana University for his undergraduate degree, graduating in 1961 before continuing at the IU School of Medicine, graduating in 1966. He entered into family medicine in Greencastle, Indiana, in 1967. He worked both as a solo physician and with a group practice.

For many years Haggerty volunteered his time teaching at the IU School of Medicine. He served as president of the Indiana Academy of Family Physicians from 1989 to 1990.

Haggerty recalls a time when other doctors did not hesitate to help out "the new kid on the block." It was an era in which young family doctors fresh out of training would search for communities in need of physicians. They were commonly warmly welcomed by the established medical community as well as the townspeople; everyone really needed their professional help.

I practiced in Greencastle for my whole career, despite the fact that I am not from there. When I was getting ready to finish medical school,

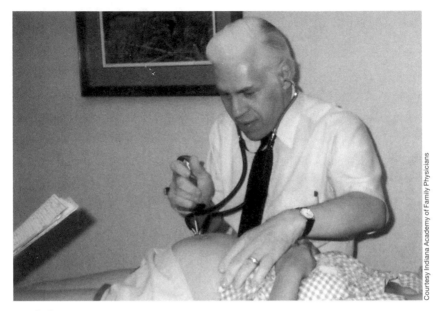

Fred Haggerty

I came to Greencastle and met three of the local doctors. They seemed nice, and they encouraged me to come, so I came. That was that.

I opened my practice on April 1, 1967, April Fools' Day. That was my first day of practice, and I believe it was on a Saturday. I had nobody scheduled or anything, of course, and I had a nurse but she and I were planning on arranging the office and getting all the logistical stuff finished up. I didn't think any patients would come. But lo and behold patients started coming in, and I actually worked until about 6:00 p.m. or 7:00 p.m. seeing patients that I had not scheduled and had no expectation of seeing. The other doctors sent them my way! Either way, I started out with a bang, and it never stopped.

But I won't lie, at first I was worried. I was happy to see the people come in that day, but all I could see was these humongous bills that I never had before in my life.

I had never before been in debt. I graduated med school without any debts. I worked the whole time I'd been at college and all through med school. I did any job I could find. If I was capable of doing it, I'd do it. I cleaned apartments. During the summers in college, I worked in a factory and at a meat shop. In med school I did the same. All the time I worked, and as a result of that I graduated without bills. That was good. Except, things changed when I came into practice—suddenly I had to buy equipment. That was a shock. I had to go into debt to buy my equipment. I bought all my stuff from the same company so I could have it all on one bill.

There's more: I had to buy a house for my family and me to live in. I had to buy a house because I couldn't find anything to rent. That would have been fine, except the only problem was I didn't even have enough money to make a down payment on the house. So wouldn't you know it? Without even knowing me, the three doctors from town who sent those patients over to me on day one cosigned the mortgage for me. I still remember them very fondly.

102

Doctor and Friend

People do not want to die alone. Haggerty's story that follows reminds us that there are extraordinary circumstances that present opportunities for doctors to confirm their friendship with patients they have grown close to over the years. Patients become friends, indeed.

Doctors will often talk about closeness to patients. There were strong, oftentimes poetic, bonds between doctors and patients back in those days. It isn't really there today, not as much anyway. There's one story in particular I can feel in my heart to this day. The patient was a lady. I suppose at the time I thought she was pretty old, but she must have been in her sixties, not older than I am today.

She was a longtime smoker with emphysema and chronic lung disease. I was helping her along for a good long while, but eventually I sent her to Indianapolis to see a specialist. He sent her back saying there wasn't anything else he could do that I wasn't already doing. So she continued to see me, and sporadically she called me. I had her on oxygen, and I would go over to her house to make a house call whenever she called me.

She had been in the hospital off and on for so many years. It just finally came to pass that she just couldn't do anything anymore. She was to a point where she would go to the hospital by ambulance and come home by ambulance. Her condition wasn't improving, and it wasn't going to. Finally she called me one night and said, "Dr. Haggerty, would you come over to the house? Please. I'm not going to make it tonight." I told her I would be right there.

When I got there, I saw she was just gasping for breath even on her oxygen—just not doing well. She was puffing away and she started gasping, trying to get some words out. She was doing everything she could do to survive, but it wasn't working. The saddest part was that I wanted to call somebody, a friend or someone in her family, but she didn't have anybody to call. So I stayed.

I did whatever I could to make her more comfortable, but nothing helped. Finally, she just said, "Well, we gave it a good run. I'm not going to be here in just a few minutes." Then just as she predicted, a few minutes later she said, "Here goes." I continued to hold her hand, and she passed on.

It just made me realize how temporary life is. I felt so close to her at that time. And it seems in that moment, I was not only her doctor but possibly her closest friend.

I continue to think about her.

103
Baby Drop

Marvin Priddy, MD, was born on July 20, 1928, and was raised in Huntington, Indiana. In 1950 he received his bachelor of science degree in anatomy and physiology from Indiana University. In 1955 he graduated from the IU School of Medicine and then continued his medical training with completion of an internship at Saint Mary Hospital, Saginaw, Michigan.

Priddy began practicing medicine in 1957, first in Bridgeport, Michigan, then with the U.S. Air Force from 1957 to 1958. After his military service, he returned to his home state of Indiana to practice in Fort Wayne. He has worked in a partnership with a scope of practice that includes general surgery, medicine, and obstetrics. He has delivered 3,800 babies in his career, which he continues today, part time, after retiring from full-time practice in 1996.

In addition to his clinical accomplishments, Priddy served as president of the Parkview Hospital medical staff and the Allen County Medical Society. He also served as chairman of the Indiana State Medical Association's delegation to the American Medical Association.

Doctors, of course, learn to think quickly in all types of circumstances. Priddy remembers how a medical student did exactly that in an uncomfortable situation:

One of the funniest things that happened to me in medical school was when we were delivering babies at the Indianapolis General Hospital [present-day Wishard Hospital]. At that hospital, most of the women were lower income and didn't have doctors of their own, so we medical students helped them out by delivering their babies.

I was delivering one baby in particular, and remember I had just finished with the delivery. There was another classmate working with me in the large delivery room. He picked up the baby to get it cleaned up and just dropped it square on its head in the pan! It went com-punk!! Right in the pan of the delivery room table. It didn't hurt the baby, but I know if it had been me, I wouldn't have known what to say in that situation at all.

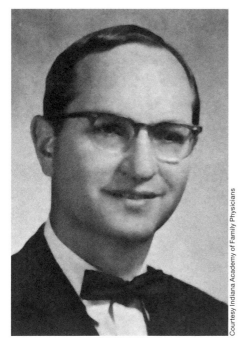

Well, I was just aghast. But my fellow doctor was able to think quickly in a potentially awkward situation. He just picked up the baby and said, "Ma'am, that's the way we wake 'em up after we deliver 'em."

Courtesy Indiana Academy of Family Physicians

Marvin Priddy

104

Protecting Little Hockey Players

Priddy explains by example that the work of a physician should extend beyond the exam room with their personal patients. It should include the broader responsibility of positively affecting the health and well-being of their local communities, states, and sometimes even nation. Priddy provides us with just one instance from his career:

There's a picture of me in the American Academy of Family Physicians' headquarters in Kansas City. I'm sewing up a local hockey player from Fort Wayne, a young man who played for the Fort Wayne Comets minor league team and eventually made it into the National Hockey League. In the photo, I look very studious and concentrated, while the hockey player has this bitter, strained grimace on his face.

Hockey players, you see, were so "tough," they would never let you inject a numbing medication into them when they got hurt. They would say, "Put the stitches in. Just do it." But in this photo, he's hurting. Oh boy, you can see it. It's written all over his face. Hockey players consider themselves really rugged and they are—they whack each other in the head like shaking hands. Or one player would hit the other over the head with a stick or a puck. One of us—Doctor [Jerry] Stuckey or I—went to almost every single Comets game as a team doctor, if we couldn't we'd get another doctor to fill in for us.

Stuckey was my partner at the time and he and I decided to try to get these guys to wear helmets. Well, they wouldn't do it. So we took a resolution to the American Medical Association when I was a delegate. The resolution said that all hockey players must wear helmets. It sounded good to us, but when the other delegates from Indiana read it they laughed and said, "That'll never happen."

So, I talked to the legal counsel for AMA and she said, "Dr. Priddy, there's no way you will get NHL [National Hockey League] players to wear helmets. But you keep pushing for this resolution." Well, that I did. She told me if I got it passed then little kids who start playing hockey in younger age groups will be forced to wear helmets, and as they graduate into higher hockey leagues they'll feel uncomfortable without wearing them.

That's exactly what happened. We got a resolution passed that required little hockey players to wear helmets, and as they got older they felt that they still wanted to have the helmets. So Jerry Stuckey and I are the fathers of hockey helmets.

105

The Recipe

Rex M. Joseph, MD, was born on February 18, 1918, and grew up in Indianapolis. He received a degree in anatomy from Indiana University, Bloomington, in 1942 and his medical degree in less than two years from the IU School of Medicine. Joseph completed an internship at Harris Memorial Methodist Hospital in Fort Worth, Texas, and a combined residency and fellowship in medicine at Indianapolis City Hospital. He always regretted the fact that he could not serve in World War II due to his 4-F classification for rheumatic fever at age fifteen.

Joseph was a company physician for Diamond Chain Company in Indianapolis beginning in 1946 and entered private practice on the south side of Indianapolis in 1948. In 1974 he folded his practice into the newly formed Saint Francis Hospital Family Practice Residency Program in Beech Grove, Indiana, and served as its clinical director until his retirement in 1980. He also received a faculty appointment in the Department of Family Medicine at the IU School of Medicine and served as medical staff president at Saint Francis and University Heights Hospitals. He died in 1985.

Joseph was the clinical director of residency during my training at Saint Francis Hospital (now Franciscan Saint Francis Health). He was a kind, jovial, and gentle man and served as a wonderful teacher and mentor to many residents during his time there.

Bartering with patients for medical services was commonplace during the golden age of family medicine. Nearly every elder family doc seems to have a story about how a patient, unable to pay with money, would offer something in exchange for his or her medical care.

Joseph's son, Rex Jr., shared this story with me about his father. It is undoubtedly one of the best bartering stories I have ever heard. However, in this case it wasn't the patient that approached the doctor, but the doctor that approached the patient and his family for something he considered more valuable than money:

The story goes that Joseph had many Italian patients on the Indianapolis south side in the late 1940s. He cared for one particular Italian family that was very poor and generally didn't have the money to pay him for his medical services. Their bill mounted to a sizable amount.

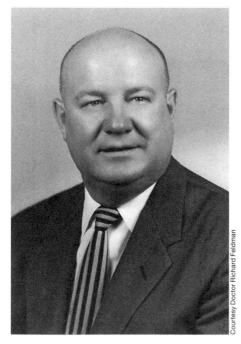

Courtesy Doctor Richard Feldman

Rex M. Joseph

One day a member of this family came in for an appointment and presented him with a gift in appreciation for his medical care—a big bowl of pasta and meatballs. It was their special family recipe. It turned out to be the best thing Joseph thought he ever ate!

So, Joseph approached the family with a proposition: He offered to forgive the entire debt, if only they would give him the recipe. They did, and it became a Joseph family tradition over the years. He would frequently make the dish when people came over for dinner, and it was always served at family get-togethers. Rex Jr. remembers as a kid how much he loved the pasta and meatballs his father would frequently cook. Even now as a vegetarian, he recalls how good those meatballs tasted.

Rex Jr. believes that his entire family and everyone who ever experienced this dish were fortunate that his father did not receive a monetary payment from that Italian family. And now he wishes to share this special recipe with the readers of this book:

Doctor Joseph's Pasta and Meatballs Sauce:

1 big pork chop (with fat)
1 piece of veal
1 piece beef round steak
(All 3 of these pieces of meat should be the same size)
Cut meat into small pieces.
Chop finely 1 clove of garlic
Brown meat and garlic in a large skillet, then add:
2 large quart cans tomatoes
2 small cans tomato paste
¼ t. oregano
Salt and pepper to taste
Cook 4-5 hours

Meatballs:

1 lb ground beef
½ lb pork sausage
¼ lb ground veal
1 clove finely chopped garlic
Pinch of oregano
Salt and pepper
1 raw egg
2 slices dry bread (leave bread out for 2 days before making meatballs)
Crumble bread into mixture
Mix all ingredients well, form into meatballs
Brown meatballs, then put into sauce about 1 hour before serving

106

Oops! An $1,800 Mistake!

Kenneth Bobb, MD, was born on February 22, 1928, and grew up in Seymour, Indiana. He received his bachelor of science in human anatomy and physiology from Indiana University in 1949 and went on to graduate from the IU School of Medicine in 1952. Bobb entered the U.S. Air Force Medical Corps in 1953 and served as a captain on active duty. After his military service, he began his practice in Seymour in 1955. For twenty-five years Bobb had a solo practice before entering into a partnership with Doctor Dan Walters. Bobb's scope of practice included general family medicine, obstetrics, and anesthesia.

Bobb received a faculty appointment in the Department of Family Medicine at the IU School of Medicine as a volunteer clinical assistant professor and also served as a board member of the Indiana State Department of Health. He served as president of the Indiana Academy of Family Physicians from 1976 to 1977.

Bobb still works in Seymour at the County Health Office as medical director of the Lutheran Community Home.

Doctors do make some mistakes. They are human after all. Bobb is sincere enough to admit that he made some during his long career. This was an error that he can chuckle about in retrospect:

Let me tell you about this gal that had a lump in her breast. She was the kind of gal you had to be careful around. She was always dressed up and wore black clothes and black bras and she used to write me notes. I never acknowledged her behavior.

One day she came in and said she had this lump. It felt like she had a breast cyst. So, I decided to aspirate it. I aspirated the area, but the needle must have missed the lump and went beside it into what I thought was a cyst. I sucked out about 20 ccs of white fluid. I didn't quite understand that, and I quit. I examined the other side, and told her she had a cyst over there and I aspirated it. The same thing from the other side! I looked at her and said, "You don't have implants do you?" She said, "I thought you knew."

I sucked out what apparently was silicone out of both breasts. I ordered a mammogram the next day that showed a crumpled up implant and the implant would have to be replaced. So, I called a plastic surgeon and told him what happened. He said that for $1,800 he would put a new implant in the left breast, which he did. If he said it would cost $5,000, I would have paid it. I wanted to make it right with the patient. I was so embarrassed. I wrote him a check for $1,800.

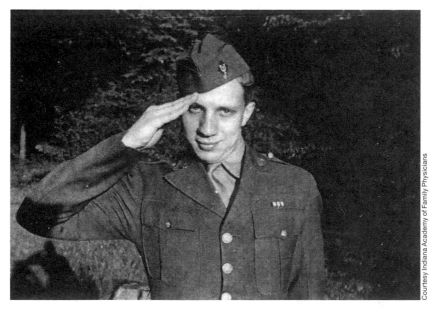

Courtesy Indiana Academy of Family Physicians

Kenneth Bobb

107

Death of a Little Boy

Encountering death and tragic situations are part of being a family doctor. As one can imagine, these difficult times affect physicians both professionally and personally. Bobb recalls a poignant moment in his career that he will never forget:

I performed a lot of anesthesia during my career. The science of anesthesia wasn't as advanced back then, and we had many more anesthetic deaths than we have today. I had a few. Fortunately today, we have better agents and technology.

I had one near death of a kid. The agent I was using was really toxic to the heart because it created a lot of ventricular arrhythmias. This kid was in for a tonsillectomy. During the surgery, he went into ventricular fibrillation, and it took us fifteen minutes to get him to turn around. I went out to talk to the family, and I told them that we weren't doing the tonsillectomy, and in fact, we didn't want him to have any surgery, ever. They were just happy to have the child alive. That boy went on a couple of years later to develop muscular dystrophy and lived until he was age thirty-two. I was his doctor all of his life.

But I remember this eight-year-old kid who had been going to the doctor for pain in his belly for two to three weeks. One afternoon, the doctor he was seeing finally decided the child had appendicitis. So, at 5:00 a.m., I got a call to my office asking me to do the anesthesia for the operation.

I went to the hospital and went to get the child. He hopped off the table onto the cart, and that didn't seem to hurt him. I thought that was odd because it would be extremely painful for someone with appendicitis to just hop off a table onto the ground. I thought to myself that he probably didn't have appendicitis. Everybody else thought he did. On the way to the operating room, I asked him what he wanted to be, and he said he didn't know. His dad was a farmer, so I asked if he wanted to be a farmer. He said, "No, I don't think so."

I said, "I bet you'll be whatever you want to be." Those were the last words that I said to that little boy. I put him to sleep and got the IV started and gave him a muscle relaxer. We were using ventilators at the time, but I didn't use one on him. When I intubated him, he started bleeding and bled a lot in his pharynx. They started the surgery and the surgery was long. It turned out he had a Burkett's lymphoma causing all that pain; it wasn't appendicitis after all. Burkett's had a high mortality rate and it was in his belly and chest.

The procedure went on for two and a half hours and I was bagging him the entire time. Nothing seemed to go well. At the end of the procedure his blood oxygen dropped, his carbon dioxide elevated, and he developed acidosis. He went into ventricular fibrillation and his heart stopped. We worked on him for an hour and never got him back.

So, all of the doctors that worked on him went to talk with the family to tell them their son had died during the procedure. It was bad. We were honest with them and told them exactly what happened, and how bad we felt about it. I told them that he had a lot of disease, that it was a long difficult procedure, and that he developed a heart rhythm problem that we couldn't fix. Certainly with a bad result, we could have been sued. Any bad result, especially in a child, might lead to that. But we had established a good relationship with the family. They were not my patients, but I knew the family and they knew me. All of that figures into it. They knew we did our best, and that we cared.

That case really got to me. I thought I wouldn't be able to do anesthesia again after that. I talked to one nurse (who is now my wife) the next day and she said, "You do so many good things for people and you have so many skills, it would be a shame for you not to continue to do your work." I went on, of course, and put it all behind me. But you never forget, and you never quite get over the tragedy of a child dying.

108

A Patient's Prayer

Bobb came to understand from many years of practicing medicine that a doctor's work is more than preventing and treating diseases. It is more than bringing a new life into the world. Helping patients and their families at the end of life is an essential part of a good doctor's responsibilities. It is part of the job, but also a portion of a career that can be very rewarding and meaningful.

I always loved becoming intimately involved with my patients and their families. They have so much respect for you that it makes you work hard to live up to their expectations.

Earlier in my career, I didn't go to my patients' funerals. My philosophy was that I had done everything I could for the patient, and once they were gone, there was nothing more I could do. But, then I realized there are things a doctor can do for the family. They are really important things. I started going to the funeral home for the visitation if I couldn't make the funeral. Hospice became a big part of my practice. There are lots of times that I go in to see a patient, and the patient is pretty much out of it, and I know there is nothing I can do for the patient. But there are things I can do for the family in helping them move on.

I enjoy being a part of people's lives and hospice, especially, gives me that opportunity. I take good care of my nursing home patients; they get so little from their caregivers and doctors. When I go to see them, I feel better.

I had one nursing home patient that had COPD [chronic obstructive pulmonary disease]. One day, as I was getting ready to leave from my visit with her she said, "The preacher was here today, but he didn't even say a prayer with me." So, I sat down and said a prayer with her. She said, "Would you mind if I said a prayer that I like?" So, she said her prayer and then every time I went back, I would try to learn that prayer from her. I wasn't doing very well learning it, and she finally wrote it out and gave it to me. I still have that prayer after all these years.

It says, "Oh God, with thankful hearts we come for family and friends and home, and for the sunshine and the rain that ripens fields of golden grain. Oh heavenly father, bless us still. We are submissive to your will. Whatever our harvests are to be, our hope, our trust, and our faith will always be in thee."

When she died she wanted me to say something at her funeral. So I used her prayer.

I have had a wonderful medical career and life. I enjoyed every bit of it.

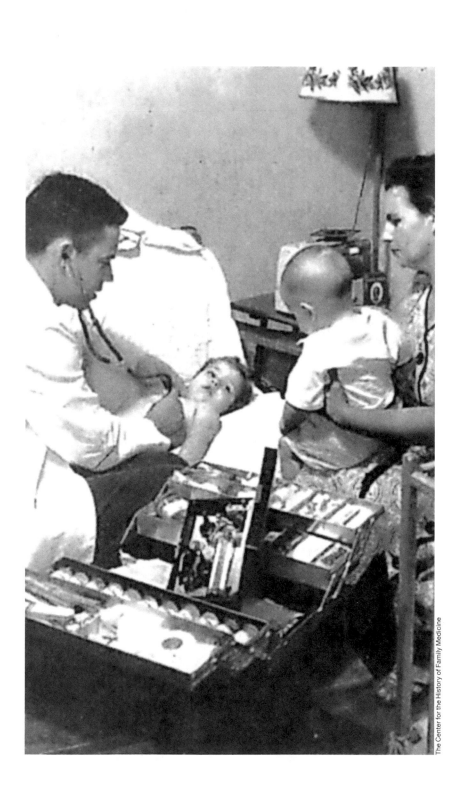

Epilogue

After a long and distinguished career, an elder family doctor related the following reflection to the author. His identity is not important because in anonymity he represents all family physicians in a commonality of emotion and belief.

As I look back over the fifty years I have been practicing, the advances are just absolutely fantastic. I can truly say that in fifty years of practice since I was welcomed into this community, I have not had one day when I hated to come to work. That doesn't mean there haven't been some challenges, but by and large, I look forward to coming to work each day. As I look back with nostalgia over the years, I think of all the friends, family, and mentors that I grew up with and have treated over the years, many of whom have passed on at this point. I consider it a great privilege and honor to have served them during this half century. I do not do OB anymore but did enjoy it when I was doing it. Now I treat children of the babies I delivered years ago and also occasionally treat their grandchildren.

What a great life and career I have had. I can't imagine being anything else in this world than what I am. I'm proud to be a family doctor.

Index